Studies in Social Policy

'Studies in Social Policy' is an important new series of textbooks intended for students of social administration and social welfare at all levels. The books are directly related to the needs of undergraduate and postgraduate students in universities, polytechnics and similar institutions as well as vocational students preparing for careers in a variety of social and other public services. The series includes the following topics:

the roles of different public and private institutions such as social services departments and building societies in meeting social needs;

introductory guides to new technical and theoretical developments relevant to the analysis of social policy such as political theory and the newly emerging specialism of the economics of social care;

contemporary social policy issues such as the use of charges in the delivery of social welfare or the problem of determining priorities in the health and personal social services.

Studies in Social Policy

Editor: Ken Judge

Published

The Building Societies
Martin Boddy

Policy-making in the National Health Service
Christopher Ham

Pricing the Social Services
Ken Judge (ed.)

Choices for Health Care
Gavin H. Mooney, Elizabeth M. Russell and Roy D. Weir

Power, Authority and Responsibility in Social Services:
Social work in area teams
Malcolm Payne

Forthcoming

The Economics of Poverty
Alan Maynard

The Economics of Social Care
Martin Knapp

Political Theory and Social Policy
Albert Weale

Policy-making in the National Health Service

A Case Study of the Leeds Regional Hospital Board

Christopher Ham

School for Advanced Urban Studies
University of Bristol

First published 1981 by
THE MACMILLAN PRESS LTD
London and Basingstoke
Associated companies in Delhi Dublin
Hong Kong Johannesburg Lagos Melbourne
New York Singapore and Tokyo

Printed in Hong Kong

British Library Cataloguing in Publication Data

Ham, Christopher
  Policy-making in the National Health Service.
  (Studies in social policy).
  1. Hospitals – England – Administration – Case studies
  2. Leeds Regional Hospital Board
  I. Title   II. Series
  362.1′09428′19   RA986

  ISBN 0–333–29137–9

To my parents

Contents

List of abbreviations

BMA	British Medical Association
DGH	District General Hospital
DHSS	Department of Health and Social Security
ENT	Ear, nose and throat
GP	General Practitioner
HAS	Hospital Advisory Service
HMC	Hospital Management Committee
JHMO	Junior Hospital Medical Officer
LGI	Leeds General Infirmary
NHS	National Health Service
RHB	Regional Hospital Board
SAMO	Senior Administrative Medical Officer
SHMO	Senior Hospital Medical Officer
TPO	Training Project Officer
WTE	Whole-time equivalent

Acknowledgements

My first debt is to the Leeds Regional Hospital Board, and its successor, the Yorkshire Regional Health Authority, for providing the financial support for the research which lies behind this study. The members and officers of the Board and the Authority, both past and present, gave freely of their time and advice, and provided the access to papers and files without which the study would not have been possible. It would be invidious to name individuals since all of those to whom I spoke have contributed something to the book, even though not all of the comments received have been incorporated into the text.

The bulk of the research was carried out between September 1975 and September 1977, when I was Research Assistant at the Nuffield Centre for Health Services Studies, University of Leeds. Thanks are due to a number of former colleagues at the Centre for reading earlier drafts of the book, in particular Mary Ann Elston and David Towell. My biggest debt, though, is to Keith Barnard, who was Research Director on the project and who acted as editorial adviser in the writing of the book. Keith has provided invaluable advice and assistance during the last four years, and there are many points in the text where his influence can be seen. Also at Leeds, Professor Arthur Taylor in the School of History supplied useful guidance and comments at a number of points during the research.

The book in its present form has been written up while I have been at the School for Advanced Urban Studies, University of Bristol. I should like to thank Michael Hill, Ruth Levitt and Randall Smith for reading an earlier draft and giving me the benefit of their comments. Also in Bristol, Ioanna Burnell provided a lot of the support needed to overcome the difficulties encountered in the last phase of writing.

Several typists made valiant attempts to cope with my writing. Special mention should be made of Olga Patchett in Leeds and Anne Merriman in Bristol.

I alone am responsible for the final text.

Bristol   CHRISTOPHER HAM
November 1979

Introduction

Issues, approaches and methods

The study which lies behind this volume was commissioned by the Leeds Regional Hospital Board on the eve of its dissolution in the spring of 1974. W. Bowring, Secretary to the Board, approached the University of Leeds's Nuffield Centre for Health Services Studies in the following terms:

> The members feel that, as the Board's activities during the period 1947–1974 will be of interest to social historians and to students of the health and social services, consideration should be given to the production of a history of the Board.

The enquiry was whether the staff of the Centre would be interested in preparing such a history. The response was unhesitatingly positive. The enquiry had been couched in terms suggesting an opportunity to prepare a genuinely critical (in the best sense) account of the first 25 years of the National Health Service (NHS) through the perspective of one of its key institutions. In other words, the Board's members were not simply seeking a conventional official history; and there has been no attempt to prepare one, but rather to accept the opportunity offered by the Board to make a contribution to the critical literature on medical care in Britain.

As the intermediary between government and the direct providers of services in each district and community, the members and officers of regional hospital boards (RHBs) were charged with making hospitals into a hospital service. Although regionalisation as a concept had been revealed in earlier blueprints for a national health service, RHBs emerged from the legislation as an innovation in public administration whose behaviour could readily arouse suspicion or provoke hostility on all sides. It was an unenviable role and one making demands of energy, insight, sense of purpose and political skill which were not readily discerned other than by those closely involved. Whatever the merits of a regional tier in the NHS today, and they continue to be argued, in the formative stage of the NHS it was to be seen as a central organisational feature. This study is a critical review of how one regional hospital board faced up to and discharged its responsibilities. By placing the work of the Board in the context of the development of the NHS as a whole, the aim has been to make more sense of the work of the Board and of the NHS.

The first concern was to consider the place that the history of the Board might have in the vast literature on medical care and the National Health Service. Other boards over the years had prepared their own histories generally as quinquennial or even annual reports, as indeed had some hospital management committees and teaching hospitals. Also, other boards had commissioned or prepared 'in-house', official histories to coincide with their formal dissolution.[1] The initial hope was that the passage of time, allied to the outsider's perspective, would enable this study to offer further insights into the working of the NHS beyond those offered by earlier histories, written, as they must have been, even more against the clock and with a consciousness that the work of the institution was not yet complete. In addition, in-house histories of any organisation are always at risk of being interpreted subsequently as 'apologias' for the decision makers, even where they avoid the more obvious danger of emerging as an unstructured 'roll-call of honour'. As a reviewer of one such history noted: 'The real need . . . is for reports suitable for judgement day rather than speech day'.[2]

Moving out from the specific field of regional hospital boards, there is no dearth of political literature on the NHS. Reports of parliamentary and departmental committees that have appeared in numbers over the years have provided a kind of running official history. The Department of Health and Social Security (DHSS) has offered its own overview through the annual reports of the Department (formerly the Ministry) and of the Chief Medical Officer. The sequence of green and white papers preceding NHS reorganisation offers a developing interpretative official history of the tripartite NHS administrative structure, while the reports, emerging from time to time from the professional bodies with an involvement in the NHS, can be seen as having quasi-official status, with the Porritt Report of 1963 on NHS structure proving to be the most influential of these. More recently, the Merrison Royal Commission has, through evidence submitted to it and the research reports it has commissioned, prompted an early assessment of the impact of reorganisation.

Academic writers have increasingly provided a wealth of literature of commentary. Social scientists, particularly health economists and medical sociologists, and latterly more management-related disciplines, such as operational research, have joined the health-related disciplines of social medicine and epidemiology in identifying for study aspects or themes of medical care and health service organisation. These academic writers, working on both large- and small-scale studies, have subjected material gathered from either primary or secondary sources to the modes of analysis offered by their particular discipline. As a result, their efforts may have lacked balance, being directed in some instances as much to the development of a discipline than to a general understanding of the NHS in its social, administrative and political context.

Despite all of these contributions, there are some important gaps in the literature. Not since Almont Lindsey's major study of the NHS to 1961[3] has there been a comprehensive history of this major public institution, while Rosemary Stevens's equally major history of the medical profession stops in the mid-1960s.[4] While there have been later essays – such as those from R. G. S. Brown, Gordon Forsyth, Brian Watkin, and Brian Abel-Smith[5] – and from the centre of decision-making, Sir George Godber, Richard Crossman, and David Owen,[6] these have not attempted to work on the same canvas. Likewise, this volume necessarily does not match the scope of the major histories working on the national scale. Nevertheless it does attempt to fill another important gap in the literature of the NHS through a close study of one institution and so to offer future historians of the Service material to illuminate and exemplify the broad sweep of development of the NHS as a major organisational innovation.

Issues and approaches

In accepting the Board's invitation to undertake a study which would be 'of interest to social historians and to students of the health and social services', it was taken as self-evident that more than a descriptive study was required. While an account of 'what the Board did' would have been of some value, an analysis of 'why the Board did what it did' seemed to offer richer opportunities for increasing our understanding of health services and health policy. More than this, it would allow various theories and concepts about policy-making to be tested in an empirical setting. Writing as a social scientist, this seemed to be a not unimportant goal. It was also taken for granted that more than a local study was required: hence the concern to use the detailed case material available on the work of the Leeds Board as an example and an illustration of the development of the NHS in its first phase. At the outset, then, the two main questions which lay behind the study were: What does the experience of the Leeds Board tell us about the dynamics of public policy? And, secondly, what does the experience of the Leeds Board tell us about the evolution of the NHS?

An answer to the second question was sought by first of all reviewing the literature on the NHS. Because this literature is extensive no more than a rapid scan was attempted. The aim of this review was to identify what seemed to be important dates, events, issues and reports. The result of this initial period of work was the identification of a number of broad themes to be investigated. These were: *planning*, particularly the development of the hospital building programme, and medical manpower planning; *collaboration*, with other health service agencies, that is local health authorities, executive councils and the boards of governors of teaching hospitals; the evolution of the so-called *'Cinderella services'* for the elderly, the mentally ill and the mentally handicapped; and the *structure of administrative control* in terms of the Board's relationship with the central department on the one hand and hospital management committees on the other. Within each theme a number of more specific questions were formulated: for example, what was the local contribution and response to the Hospital Plan? How did the distribution of medical staff within the region change during the period? Through what channels did the Board relate to local health authorities? What priority was given to services for the mentally ill? What was the impact of the Hospital Advisory Service? What was the nature of the Board's relationship with the central department?

The initial literature review, together with an assessment of the most practicable research strategy, led to an examination of these themes not continuously throughout the years 1947–74, but within four time periods: 1947–53, which was bounded by the establishment of boards as shadow authorities and the appointment of the Guillebaud Committee to review the cost and operation of the NHS; 1953–60, which saw the NHS structure emerge untouched from the Guillebaud review, and increasing acceptance of the service by both major political parties; 1960–7, the era of optimism and expansion founded on the building programme with its vision of a hospital service fit for the next century and the emergent management ideology which reflected the spirit of the times; and, lastly, 1967–74, when the structure of the NHS came under much critical scrutiny and the prolonged debate on reorganisation ended with the demise of the Board but the preservation of the regional tier.

In its first draft the history of the Board followed this pattern. A chapter was devoted to each of these periods, and within chapters the themes of planning, collaboration, the Cinderella services and the structure of administrative control were discussed. An attempt was thus made to blend thematic and chronological analysis, the emphasis being slightly more on the latter than the former. On completion of the first draft progress was reviewed and it was decided to reverse this emphasis. By then it was clear that the sense of continuity of issues which resulted from a thematic presentation outweighed the sense of inter-connectedness of issues and events which is the major advantage of a chronological approach: hence the thematic structure of this book, which is organised into four parts.

The first part establishes the context and the setting, with Chapter 1 outlining the background to the NHS and providing an overview of its development in the first phase, and Chapter 2 describing the Leeds Region and the way in which the Leeds Board went about organising its work. The second part discusses the Board's activities as a planning and policy-making agency, with Chapter 3 concentrating on hospital building and the capital programme, Chapter 4 examining medical staffing, and Chapter 5 long-stay services and their development. The third part looks at the Board's work in a wider context, with Chapter 6 focusing on hospital services in the city of Leeds, where policy-making was complicated by the presence of a teaching hospital run by a separate board of governors, Chapter 7 considering liaison between hospital authorities and other health service agencies, and Chapter 8 looking at the relationship between the Board and the central department. Finally, the fourth part seeks to draw out general lessons from the study for the NHS.

As well as seeking to relate the experience of the Leeds RHB to the NHS as a whole, an attempt has been made to examine the contribution of the data to the growing interest in the study of public policy. In order to do this some framework was needed to guide the analysis. However, the study of public administration and public policy, and indeed of social administration and social policy, though not in their infancy, are still far from the stage where they are able to offer a ready-made theoretical framework for work such as this. In searching and researching the literature, which, as is explained below, extended right through the period of research and writing-up, there seemed a clear case for 'intellectual pluralism'.[7] Put another way, it was decided to draw on a number of disciplines and strands of work in attempting to make sense of the policy-making activities of the Board. Brown, in a similar context, has made the following case for adopting this approach:

> We shall probably find it best to use different tools for different purposes, as a market gardener puts different attachments on his rotovator for different stages in the process of preparing the soil, hoeing and harvesting his crops.[8]

The tools we initially used were, for obvious reasons, those with which we were most familiar. Thus Ham, a political scientist by background, and with an immediate past interest in the operation of pressure groups in the British political system, on which, interestingly, Eckstein's study of the British Medical Association (BMA) was for many years a standard text,[9] brought to the research an interest in exploring the dynamics of power and decision-making. Given the paucity of work on local political systems in the United Kingdom, Ham was particularly keen to examine the applicability of the kinds of approaches used by American political scientists like Dahl and Bachrach and Baratz.[10] At a minimum this implied looking at whose will prevailed and whose interests were served by decision-making and non-decision-making processes. Barnard shared these concerns, and, as an historian with a special interest in health planning and the operation of planning systems, he brought another dimension to the research. Indeed, half-way through the period of full-time research Barnard became co-director of another project examining the operation of the NHS planning system introduced in March 1976. These additional commitments meant that Barnard's involvement became that of editorial adviser; hence the sole authorship of this book by Ham.

These tools were sharpened, refined and added to as the research progressed. Two main influences were at work here. First, in the process of gathering data it became clear that the tools were inadequate. This applied in particular to the data presented in the third part on the Board's relationship with other organisations. To give an example, as data were unearthed about the interaction between the Board and the central department it became necessary to examine more closely the literature on central–local relationships for hints on how to interpret the information which was gathered. Or again, in trying to understand collaboration between the Board and other health service agencies, help was sought from the literature on inter-organisational relationships in the health policy field. The second influence was Ham's developing interest and knowledge, in particular in the literature from the growing area of policy analysis. This point requires a little elaboration.

Policy analysis is susceptible to a number of different interpretations, but a distinction can be made between analysis *for* policy and analysis *of* policy.[11] It is the latter which is of concern here, and the analysis of policy encompasses both the analysis of policy determination and the analysis of policy content. Now, the analysis of policy determination is in part to do with detailed examination of policy and decision-making processes, and in part it is concerned with the distribution of power. Thus, as well as making use of a body of work often termed decision theory, which seeks to explain decision-making in terms of the two dominant models of rationality and incrementalism, it draws on power theories such as élitism and pluralism. There is some linking of power theory and decision theory in the work of Graham Allison, who has argued that there are three models which can be used to understand policy-making processes.[12] There is, first, the familiar rational actor model, which sees actions as being performed by purposeful agents with certain goals and objectives. These agents have to choose between alternative courses of action in order to achieve these goals. Alternatives are assumed to have a set of consequences attached, and rational choice consists of selecting that alternative whose consequences rank highest. Secondly, there is the organisational process model which sees action not as rational choice, but as the output of organisational behaviour. This behaviour is largely the enactment of established routines in which sequential attention is given to goals and standard operating procedures are adopted. In contrast, the bureaucratic politics model sees action neither as choice nor output but rather as the resultant of bargaining between groups and individuals in the political system.

All of these tools from the policy analysis literature were found to be useful additions to those which were available at the outset. They were particularly helpful in making sense of the data presented in the second part. In analysing these data on policy-making processes, it was found to be illuminating to ask the following questions: what approach to policy-making was adopted? Who was involved? How was the problem or issue defined? What was the policy response? How was the policy implemented? Who benefited? And whose will prevailed? This is similar to the approach used by Rudolf Klein to analyse health policy-making, and Klein's work was an encouragement in this study.[13] There have been few attempts to understand health policy from a policy analysis perspective, but those studies, like Klein's, which have been undertaken suggest there are further insights to be gained from this perspective. Again, the related social policy work of Heclo,[14] Higgins,[15] and Hall and her colleagues,[16] which has been reviewed elsewhere,[17] has pointed the way for future studies.

This brief glance at the menu is intended only as a guide to the later courses. The main point being made is that, contrary to what manuals on research methods would have us believe, there is no neat progression in research from literature review to hypothesis generation to hypothesis testing to the writing-up of results. The reality is much messier, and in this case there was a continuous interchange between theory and data, and data and theory. As has been explained, the initial framework was modified (hopefully improved) over time, and there was a continual return to the literature for guidance on what was discovered. In doing this, it is hoped that the danger of *post hoc* rationalisation has been avoided.

Research methods

The questions asked about the Board's activities have now been set out, and the next task is to explain how data on these activities were gathered. The primary data were of two sorts: documentary sources, and oral and, in a few cases, written evidence from former members and officers of the Board, and others closely involved in its work.

Given the constraints of time and money within which the research was conducted, an early decision was made to concentrate on the official minutes of the Board and its major committees. The justification for doing so was summed up nicely by a former officer who described the minutes as the 'authority', and as such the definitive record on which the work should be based (this officer was the only person approached who refused to be interviewed). Most of the time was in fact spent examining the minutes of the Board and its Finance and General Purposes Committee,[18] to whom all of the other committees of the Board reported. A judgement was made that any issues of significance would find their way to the Board or this Committee, and could thereby be traced back to source. Interviews were used to check whether any issues considered by the interviewees to be important had in fact been missed.

Rather less time was spent examining the minutes of a small number of other committees: the Mental Health and Geriatrics Committee,[19] the Specialist Services Advisory Committee, the Staff and Establishments Committee, the Works and Buildings Committee, and the Regional Liaison Committee. Occasional reference was made to other committees like the Selection Committee and the Nursing Services Committee; while the minutes of some committees, like the Advisory Committee on Anglican Chaplains and the Regional Rheumatism Committee, were not consulted at all. It was found that the bound minute books usually contained background reports and papers presented to Board members, but, where they did not, file copies were asked for and received. Sometimes these were major planning reports too large to be appended to the minutes, like the Board's submission to the Hospital Plan, which because of the colour of its cover and its size was known as the 'green goddess'; and sometimes they were confidential documents like the reports of the Hospital Advisory Service. Other documentary sources like statistical reviews of the Region and the Board's annual accounts were also drawn on. Very occasionally, internal memoranda and files on particular issues were examined. The development of the new hospital at Eastburn, described in Chapter 2, was a case in point. Unfortunately, time did not permit the examination of outside documentary sources like local and regional newspapers.

A central methodological problem involved in this kind of historical research is that of selectivity. The reasons why the minutes of the Board and its Finance and General Purposes Committee were selected for attention at the expense of other committees has already been explained. The second aspect of selectivity is what to look for, and not look for, in the minutes which are examined. Here the research was guided by two considerations: first, since one aim was to look at what the experience of the Leeds Board tells us about the development of the NHS, a number of issues, events and themes worthy of investigation were identified. Hence, as was explained above, questions like, 'what was the Board's contribution and response to the Hospital Plan?' were asked. (Since the research was also concerned to shed light on policy-making processes, other questions were asked, including what approach to planning was used, who was involved, what was the policy response, how was the policy implemented, and so on.) The second consideration was what issues occupied the attention of the Board? Thus those issues which the Board itself selected were chosen for discussion and analysis. For the most part these coincided with what was expected to be found on the basis of the previous identification of issues: the Board did indeed spend a lot of time on planning issues, there was a major concern with new building, and so on. But some issues arose in the minutes which had not been anticipated: the case of the consultant anaesthetist described in Chapter 8 is an example, and the extent to which hospital services in Leeds occupied the Board's time is another.

It might be argued that this approach neglects the importance of non-issues, and issues which do not get on to the agenda.[20] It might be said too that the method of selection emphasises policy-making and change at the expense of policy maintenance, which some see as being the major task of public agencies.[21] The second point is fully accepted, and the research showed that most of the Board's time was spent maintaining existing policies and continuing established procedures and practices. Only rarely were new policies discussed, and even more rarely were they accepted. This is where an attempt is made to shed light on the non-decision-making thesis, since non-decision-making does actually involve taking decisions. The important point is that these are decisions to resist change and maintain the *status quo*. Many examples of such decisions are given in the following chapters. Nevertheless, it is acknowledged that the method used here does not permit an analysis of what issues are kept off the agenda, because by definition the examination of minutes is concerned only with the agenda. To some extent this could have been investigated by means of the interviews undertaken, and in part this was attempted. But whether because of the haziness of memories or the distance of the time people were asked to recollect, the interviews did not succeed in throwing up major issues which the Board failed to consider or which were suppressed by other means. Most of the interviews took place after the interviewees had read earlier draft chapters. The items discussed at these interviews were many and varied, although structured around the drafts. At some point in each interview, the interviewer asked if any significant issues had not been covered or if the Board itself had failed to pay sufficient attention to important issues in the region. Only in the case of the Cinderella services did some of the interviewees confirm what had already been identified from the documentary sources – that these services did not receive the priority which their conditions seemed to warrant. This is discussed further in Chapter 5.

It is worth mentioning briefly another problem involved in the research method, that of the accuracy of the documentary sources and the means of interpretation. Despite Crossman's warnings about the veracity of the Cabinet minutes,[22] the minutes consulted have been accepted as an accurate official record – the 'authority' – of the Board's work. This view has been reinforced by the very few occasions on which Board members sought to amend the minutes. The minutes were full enough to enable a narrative account of the Board's activities to be constructed, and this was then used as a basis for the interviews. It was at this point, when the evidence from the documentary sources came into contact with people's memories, that the significance of interpretation entered in. Most of those interviewed accepted that the researchers had better access to the documents of the time and therefore had the 'facts' at hand with which they could not quarrel. But the way the facts were interpreted was more problematic: hence the value of the oral and written evidence of the interviewees.

Two consequences followed. First, because the minutes were written by the lay administrative staff, and because, as is explained in the following chapter, relationships between these staff and the medical administrative staff were sometimes strained, due account had to be taken of possible biases in the minutes. As one of the interviewees (himself a medical administrator) warned, the problem was not so much that the minutes were inaccurate but that they did not necessarily tell the whole story. Or, as another medical administrator put it after reading an earlier draft:

It may well be that the natural bias towards lay administration of the minutes which were drafted by the secretariat has resulted in your lack of appropriate recognition of the medical effort in these early years when most of the Board's work was concerned with matters of purely medical import.

The response to these points was to take seriously the evidence of those interviewed.

The second consequence was to question the implicit positivist assumption that it was possible to write 'a history' of 'the Board'. The longer the research continued, the more it became apparent that there was not one but several histories or competing interpretations of the Board's activities. It was about this time that the importance of Carrier and Kendall's critique of studies of social policy which seek 'the one "correct reading of events" '[23] became clear. As Carrier and Kendall suggest, it seems wise to prepare 'a range of plausible accounts', and, where the strength of the material will stand this kind of analysis, this has been attempted.

A connected point repeatedly stressed by the interviewees was that the early drafts, based as they were on the documentary sources alone, lacked 'flavour' because they did not give sufficient attention to the effect of individuals on the Board's work. As one former officer wrote:

Ultimately I suppose you are writing the history of the Leeds Regional Hospital Board which is in a sense a *non sequitur* in that the Board was ultimately the sum of the characters who made it up and the system clearly would not tolerate that sort of history.

This coincided with the reading of Graham Allison's critique of those who use the rational actor model of explanation, and especially his point that this model often sees government, or in this case the Board, as a unitary actor rationally seeking to maximise satisfactions in the pursuit of goals and objectives.[24] It was recognised that this was one of the implicit assumptions in the initial stages of the research, and the early drafts which resulted. Building on Allison's insight, the later work attempted to correct this assumption by taking account of the diversity of 'the Board' as well as the range of interpretations of its activities. There remained the problem of language, and, while not seeking to reify 'the Board', continued use has been made of this designation where a more specific term — for example, the Board's officers, the chairman, the secretary — is inappropriate, usually to denote action on its behalf or decisions of the full Board or its committees.

The interviews which were conducted took place throughout the whole period. In all, 35 people were interviewed, some on more than one occasion. The biggest group of these, 15 in total, were former officers, divided almost equally between lay and medical administrative staff. Both of the Senior Administrative Medical Officers (SAMOs) were interviewed at length, as was the sole surviving secretary. The next biggest group comprised former members, including a former chairman, and this totalled six people, again fairly evenly divided between lay and medical members. The remaining interviewees came from a variety of backgrounds, the largest identifiable group being doctors and lay administrators concerned with hospital services in the city of Leeds. This group also included two hospital management committee secretaries, a consultant psychiatrist, a consumer group representative, an academic who had been involved in various ways in developments in the Region, and two people with experience at senior levels in the Ministry of Health and DHSS. There are some obvious gaps in this list — for example, financial, nursing and architectural staff of the Board — but again within the resources available it was impossible to be comprehensive in coverage. It was mentioned earlier that only once was an interview refused, by a former lay officer who took the view that the documentary sources provided sufficient evidence for the research.

The interviews were held in people's homes, offices or our offices. All of the interviews were conducted by Ham, on a few occasions with assistance from Barnard. The interviews were semi-structured, with in most cases a draft chapter or chapters forming the basis of the discussion. As far as possible an easy conversational style was adopted, though always in the knowledge that there were certain issues that had to be covered in the time available (which varied from 30 minutes to three hours). At least once, and usually more often, interviewees were given the opportunity to raise issues they felt were important and had not been touched on either in the drafts or in conversation.

A tape recorder was used in the initial interviews, but the time needed to transcribe tapes proved prohibitive; hence in later interviews note-taking was relied on. A subsidiary reason for rejecting tapes was an unease among many of the early interviewees at the presence of a recorder, coupled with not infrequent requests that the 'machine' be turned off while 'off-the-record' information was communicated. Like Heclo and Wildavsky in their interviews with ministers and civil servants,[25] the value of building up a stock of information and stories to trade in return for further information was quickly learned. Similarly, the private language of the interviewees became familiar and in this way the researchers were more readily accepted. Of course, much of the data gathered through interviews cannot be used because it is libellous, uncorroborated or simply irrelevant; and because too great a concern with personal details, however interesting to those closely involved, may lack relevance to a wider audience. In any case, oral history, like the written record, is not intended to reveal all, and is prey to the distortions of time, selective recall and retrospective order. No doubt those interviewed will not always agree with the account which follows, especially when their evidence has been interpreted in ways other than those of their choosing. When judgement has been passed, it has been on the basis of the various evidence available and recognising the limitations of both official records and oral history. In this respect the researcher is in a privileged and unique position, having access to many different accounts of the same event. The research has tried to remain faithful to these accounts, even if they have not always been used. Careful readers will doubtless recognise another history – the sort 'the system would not tolerate', as one of the interviewees expressed it – striving chrysalis-like to break through.

In the final chapter an attempt has been made to identify the lessons which can be drawn from the study. As has been said many times, there are limits to the generalisability of case studies, though the value of comparative case studies has been highlighted by recent work.[26] This is not such a work. Rather, it is a study of one institution through which it is hoped to illuminate and exemplify various aspects of the development of the NHS, and test certain ideas in currency in the policy analysis literature. The richness of detail is perhaps the main contribution which the study makes to the literature on the NHS, and it is hoped that others will want to take some of the ideas presented here and apply them in prospective studies. It is also anticipated that health service practitioners who read the following pages will on more than one occasion experience a sense of *déjà vu*, if not *plus ça change* . . . There may well be lessons to learn from the past, and it seems no more than ordinarily prudent to make use of historical intelligence in laying plans for the future. Moreover, several academic writers have begun to show an interest in learning in the policy process,[27] and although this line of analysis has not been pursued here it may be that data from the study have something to contribute to this debate.

Finally, a word about the audience to whom the book is addressed: in reporting the data presented here I have had in mind more than the simple dichotomy of on the one hand the customer, the Board (in practice its successor, the Regional Health Authority), and, on the other hand, academic colleagues. I have been conscious that the study may be relevant to those involved in the NHS, whether as members or officers, and whether in the Leeds Region or outside; to academic colleagues, whether in departments of social administration or in departments of political science; and to students, whether seeking an understanding of health services and public policy, or about to undertake similar research. Since the main body of the book seeks to blend description and analysis, data and theory, and local and national material, it is not possible to follow Allison,[28] and to direct readers to one chapter or another. With the exception of this introduction, which I anticipate will mainly interest the research student, and the following chapter, which is meant for those unfamiliar with the history of the NHS, I have tried throughout to write for all potential readers.

1

Background and Overview: the Creation and Evolution of the NHS

The hospital and specialist services that existed in England and Wales in 1948 were the product of private charity, municipal endeavour and war-time exigency. Private charity had produced the voluntary hospitals, which ranged from the large teaching hospitals, having the benefit of modern equipment and a full complement of consultant staff, to the small cottage hospitals, usually staffed by general practitioners, and lacking all but the most essential facilities. In all, the NHS took control of 1145 voluntary hospitals with 90 000 beds on the 5 July 1948.[1]

Municipal endeavour had resulted in the evolution of institutions of even greater contrast: some local authorities had taken advantage of the permissive powers of the 1929 Local Government Act and consequently had been able to provide large general hospitals of a standard approaching that of the best voluntary hospitals; other councils had not been as progressive, and still maintained the former poor law hospitals, public assistance institutions and workhouses, much as they had always been. In addition, all county and county borough councils possessed a variety of special hospitals, including those for the treatment of infectious diseases, tuberculosis, and mental illness and deficiency. On the appointed day, 1545 municipal hospitals with 390 000 beds were taken over.[2]

Finally, there was the legacy of the war-time emergency hospital scheme, in the form of hutted annexes, and, in some cases, entire hutted hospitals, which had been constructed in anticipation of large civilian and military casualties. These were usually to be found in the grounds of existing local authority hospitals and institutions, and some 52 000 beds had been added to the country's hospital resources in this way. Also, during the war, many other hospitals had been improved and upgraded by the addition of operating theatres, the provision of new equipment and the like.[3]

The patchwork of hospitals which had resulted from these three sources left much to be desired. During the war, the Ministry of Health had commissioned a number of regional surveys covering the whole country, and these surveys are a mine of information for the historian.[4] They showed first that there was a shortage of beds, and that this problem was compounded by maldistribution. Nationally, it was estimated that about one-third more beds was needed. In the Yorkshire region, the hospital surveyors calculated that, in 1938, there was a deficiency of 7052 beds for acute, maternity, tuberculosis, infectious diseases and chronic sick cases. Yet this regional figure obscured even greater inequalities within the region. While overall there were 6.6 beds per thousand of population, in Harrogate there were 10.7 and in Dewsbury and York only 5.5.[5] Clearly, some sections of the population had much better access to hospital beds than others.

This applied equally with regard to staffing, and the shortage and maldistribution of specialists was the second major deficiency of the pre-war hospital system. The Yorkshire surveyors stated that:

> the number of properly trained and experienced specialists now in the region is inadequate for the population to be served. This is not so much a criticism as a simple statement of fact, but it is obvious that, to serve a fully efficient hospital service, the supply of consultants will have to be materially increased.[6]

Again this shortcoming was made worse by the way in which the consultants working in the region were distributed. Of the 120 'pure' specialists employed in Yorkshire, 48 were located in Leeds and 25 in Bradford, with only 5 in Huddersfield and none at all in Dewsbury.[7] Consultants from the main urban centres did, however, visit other hospitals in the region, and Dewsbury and District General Infirmary, to take one example, had the services of 10 visiting physicians and surgeons of consultant status. The surveyors considered this to be a good hospital which 'appears to meet the local demand fairly well since the waiting list is *nil* on the medical side, and runs from 20 to 50 on the surgical side, exclusive of cases of tonsils and adenoids'[8] (original emphasis). On the other hand, the overall shortage of staff meant that many of the small cottage hospitals, which supposedly were able to call on specialists when required, often had to rely on local general practitioners, and in one such institution it was found that 'practically all of the work of the hospital is done by the general practitioner staff, except in very special cases'. The surveyors recommended that 'in reorganisation, arrangements should be made so that the conduct of the surgical and other specialist work of the hospital is the function and responsibility of the visiting consultants'.[9]

Unfortunately, the shortage and maldistribution of beds and consultants was not helped by the disorganised state of the hospital and specialist services. The fact that there were two different forms of hospital ownership, private and public, and within these two forms the presence of numerous, largely autonomous authorities — county councils, county borough councils, and the boards of voluntary hospitals — effectively precluded attempts to plan comprehensively for the needs of patients, and militated against coordination, co-operation and collaboration. Indeed, many commentators go as far as to deny the existence of any one hospital 'system'.[10] One writer even contends that 'irrational organisation . . . was, in many ways, the most serious fault of the pre-Health Service medical system'.[11] Disorganisation led to unhealthy competition between the municipal and voluntary sectors and unnecessary duplication of services. In Yorkshire, the surveyors wished to express 'as strongly as may be their opinion that no effective or economic hospital organisation can be provided in any given district unless the fullest co-operation between the two hospital systems is, in fact, developed'.[12] And only in Leeds, where a Joint Hospitals Advisory Committee had been formed in 1936, did they find such co-operation to be practised. Elsewhere there was much work to be done: with the judicious use of the double negative, the surveyors observed that in Bradford 'the Royal Infirmary has not been able to get a definite relationship [with the local authority] created but the attitude is not unfriendly';[13] and in Halifax they recommended that 'co-operation between the Halifax Royal Infirmary and the Halifax General Hospital should be improved'.[14]

One cause of friction between the voluntary and municipal hospitals had traditionally been that the former concentrated on the more interesting acute cases, leaving the latter to deal with chronic and long-stay patients. In summarising the hospital surveys, the Nuffield Provincial Hospitals Trust noted that 'it is for the provision for the chronic sick that the surveyors reserve their bitterest comments'.[15] This was certainly true of Yorkshire, where the surveyors stated: 'There is, perhaps, no side of hospital provision which has given rise to more disquiet of mind on the part of the surveyors than the provision made for the chronic sick.' They went on to record that, 'almost without exception, the accommodation for the chronic sick is made in public assistance hospitals', and recommended a 'complete and revolutionary change' in the care of these patients.[16] Among their proposals was the suggestion that all chronic cases should be first sent to a general hospital; but to effect this change, and others like it, it was becoming increasingly apparent that the old order of hospital ownership, management and organisation would have to be overturned.

The creation of the National Health Service

Although the deficiencies which have just been described were recognised before 1939, it was the experience of the Second World War which made the demand for change more widespread and which eventually resulted in the passage of the National Health Service Act in 1946. As Abel-Smith has noted, 'the War was a major educative experience not only for the Ministry but also for the top doctors and many middle-class patients'.[17] The Emergency Medical Service which was created in 1939 and which included the Emergency Hospital Scheme, revealed to senior consultants the sad state of the country's smaller hospitals. Civil servants and politicians quickly accepted that when peacetime conditions returned something would have to be done about the organisation and financing of hospitals. Thus the Minister of Health announced in October 1941 that after the War a comprehensive *hospital* service would be provided. Just over a year later the Beveridge Report was published, following which the Government announced its acceptance of the idea of a comprehensive *health* service as recommended in the Report. In February 1944 a White Paper containing the Government's suggestions for 'a National Health Service'[18] was issued, and discussions with interested groups were then seriously begun. But just when it seemed that some measure of agreement had been reached, the Labour Party was voted into office at the 1945 general election and Aneurin Bevan replaced Henry Willink as Minister of Health. Bevan published his

National Health Service Bill in March 1946 and it became law in November of the same year.

In the five-year debate preceding the Act the two main problems concerning hospitals were how to marry the municipal and voluntary hospitals, and what form of organisational structure to introduce. The first firm Government proposals on these issues appeared in the 1944 White Paper, which suggested that joint boards should be established to administer local authority hospitals, while voluntary hospitals should remain independent. The joint boards would plan the hospital and specialist services of their areas and enter into contractual arrangements with voluntary hospitals where necessary.

These suggestions were substantially modified after Willink had had discussions with the parties concerned. In the Minister's revised plan of 1945, councils and voluntary bodies were to continue to run their own institutions, and at area level there would be joint planning boards containing representatives of local authorities and voluntary hospitals. Parallel to these boards the Minister proposed to set up area planning councils for other health services, and above these there were to be approximately 10 regional planning authorities. This plan has variously been described as 'a masterpiece in the art of compromise'[19] and 'a somewhat clumsy structure',[20] but there can be little doubt that, in seeking to gain the approval of the pressure groups most affected, Willink had devised an extremely complicated solution. Essentially, he had arrived at this point as a result of trying to reconcile what have been termed 'probably two incompatibles – the independence of the voluntary hospitals and a co-ordinated hospital service'.[21]

It was at this point that Aneurin Bevan entered the debate. Faced with the same problem, the answer Bevan put forward was nothing less than the appropriation of voluntary hospitals. However, the Minister rejected local government control of the hospital service because

> when I considered what to do with the voluntary hospitals when they had been taken over, and who was to receive them, I had to reject the local government unit, because the local authority area is no more an effective gathering ground for the patients of the hospitals than the voluntary hospitals themselves.

Instead, he decided 'to create an entirely new hospital service, to take over the voluntary hospitals, and to take over the local government hospitals and to organise them as a single hospital service'.[22] In this way he was able to marry the voluntary and municipal hospitals.

Once this problem had been solved, the question of organisational structure had to be tackled. Bevan told MPs that investigations had shown that

> the effective hospital unit should be associated with the medical school. If you grouped the hospitals in about 16 to 20 regions around the medical schools, you would then have within those regions the wide range of disease and disability which would provide the basis for your specialised hospital service.[23]

Thus the Minister proposed to establish regional hospital boards, appointed after consultation with various bodies including local authorities, the voluntary hospitals, the medical profession and the medical schools, to plan and administer the hospitals in each region, these regions to be based on teaching hospitals. And, since some form of regional administration was favoured by the doctors, and had been shown to work during the war, this proposal caused very little controversy. Beneath the regional boards, management committees, appointed by the boards themselves, would be responsible for the day-to-day administration of a hospital or a group of hospitals in accordance with the regional plan.

However, Bevan was not being strictly accurate when he referred to 'a single hospital service', for the teaching hospitals on which the regions were centred were to be separately administered by boards of governors. These boards were to be allowed, unlike the regional hospital boards, to retain control of the endowments of their hospitals. This was just one of the concessions Bevan made in an effort to gain the support of consultants for his bill. Other concessions included the decision to allow pay beds in NHS hospitals; to permit consultants to opt for a part-time NHS contract leaving time for private work; and to create a system of distinction awards for consultants of exceptional ability. It was these moves that led Bevan to say of consultants that he had 'stuffed their mouths with gold'.[24]

Under the 1946 Act it was the Minister's duty 'to promote the establishment in England and Wales of a comprehensive health service designed to secure improvement in the physical and mental health of the people of England and Wales and the prevention, diagnosis, and treatment of illness'. This comprehensive health service was divided into three parts for the purpose of administration. Hospital and specialist services were to be administered in the manner already described; general medical and dental services, pharmaceutical services and supplementary ophthalmic services became the responsibility of executive councils; and health centres, ambulance services, health visiting, midwifery and sundry other services became the responsibility of local health authorities.

Under Section 12 of the Act, regional hospital boards were given the duty 'generally to administer on behalf of the Minister the hospital and specialist services provided in their area'. These terms of reference were later amplified by ministerial regulations and circulars. From these it became clear that the Minister intended to give boards a large measure of autonomy. Although they would be acting as his agents, he wanted them 'to feel from the outset . . . a lively sense of independent responsibility'.[25] Their main functions were in the fields of planning and administration. To quote from an early circular, the general organisation and supervision of services

> comprises the main activities and responsibilities of the Regional Boards. It is under this head that the Boards will operate as the bodies responsible to the Minister for what may be termed the strategy of the services in their area, for reviewing and assessing the resources of the service, planning the best use of them and determining the contribution to be made by each hospital or group, working out developments of the service, and giving general oversight to the operations of the Hospital Management Committees.[26]

Although not required to submit formal plans to the Ministry, boards were expected to survey the facilities at their disposal in order to identify 'the gaps to be filled and the needs to be met'.[27] As part of this process, they had to determine the use of hospitals, appoint and deploy senior medical and dental staff, and organise a programme of capital works. In addition, they had to ensure that the actions of hospital management committees did not conflict with the strategic plans worked out at regional level.

These management committees stood in the same relationships to boards as did the latter to the Minister: that is, while they were the boards' agents, it was stressed that 'the Minister wants these

Committees to enjoy the maximum of autonomy in regard to local day-to-day administration, reserving power to the Boards to decide questions of wider policy, to control major building operations, to approve the Committees' budgets and other similar functions'.[28] In short, hospital management committees were to be responsible for the more routine aspects of administration, leaving regional boards free to exercise overall planning and supervisory functions.

Thus it was Bevan who piloted the Bill through Parliament and who was Minister when the National Health Service came into operation on 5 July 1948. With characteristic eloquence, Bevan explained the guiding philosophy behind the NHS in the following words:

> The collective principle asserts that the resources of medical skill and the apparatus of healing shall be placed at the disposal of the patient, without charge, when he or she needs them; that medical treatment and care should be a communal responsibility; that they should be made available to rich and poor alike in accordance with medical need and by no other criteria. It claims that financial anxiety in time of sickness is a serious hindrance to recovery, apart from its unnecessary cruelty. It insists that no society can legitimately call itself civilised if a sick person is denied medical aid because of lack of means.[29]

Although his predecessors had laid the groundwork for the NHS, Bevan made a major personal contribution both to the principle that access to health care should be available to *all* on grounds of medical need and not ability to pay, rather than 90 per cent of the population as some had suggested, and also to the administrative machinery which was established. Nevertheless, Bevan recognised that there were defects in his grand design, not least the fact that the members of hospital boards and committees and executive councils were selected and not elected, and he expressed the hope that a future re-organisation of local government would enable hospitals to be brought under the control of elected local authorities.[30] As we shall see, this was a debate that was to surface 20 years later.

The NHS up to 1974

In the years immediately after 1948 the NHS seemed to be in an almost permanent state of financial crisis. The original calculations of the cost of the Service prepared by Beveridge and the Ministry of Health were based on incomplete information and were soon found to be underestimates. Supplementary estimates were therefore necessary in 1948/1949 and 1949/1950, and an expenditure ceiling was imposed in March 1950. A year later charges were introduced to help meet the cost, thus provoking the resignation of Aneurin Bevan, who by that time was Minister of Labour, and two junior ministers, including a later Prime Minister, Harold Wilson.

It was soon realised that the Beveridge assumption that there was a fixed quantity of illness which a state medical service would successfully reduce, thereby causing costs to level out after a number of years, was a fallacy. The assumption had some validity with regard to spectacles and dentures, where demand was particularly high immediately after July 1948, but in respect of other services it was gradually appreciated that demand (if not need) was virtually unlimited.

Nevertheless, the view persisted that the NHS was not making good use of the available resources, and so in May 1953 the Government appointed the Guillebaud Committee,

to review the present and prospective cost of the National Health Service, to suggest means, whether by modifications in organisation or otherwise, of ensuring the most effective control and efficient use of such Exchequer funds as may be made available; to advise how, in view of the burdens on the Exchequer, a rising charge upon it can be avoided while providing for the maintenance of an adequate Service; and to make recommendations.[31]

The Committee's report was published in 1956, and it found that there was no evidence that the Service had been extravagant or grossly inefficient. Indeed, on the basis of work carried out by Brian Abel-Smith and Richard Titmuss, the Committee drew attention to the fact that the cost of the NHS as a proportion of gross national product had in fact fallen from 3.75 per cent in 1949/1950 to 3.25 per cent in 1953/1954.[32] As far as the organisation of the NHS was concerned, the Committee was against any change, arguing that more time was needed before a proper assessment could be made. While the tripartite structure was acknowledged to have caused 'undeniable problems',[33] in the Committee's view this was because 'habits of co-operation need time to grow and, insofar as they are at present weak, we believe that the cause lies in the newness of the Service, rather than in any organisational weakness'.[34]

The generally clean bill of health given by the Guillebaud Committee was reiterated in a series of reports published by the Acton Society Trust between 1955 and 1959.[35] The Committee and the Trust agreed that, if there were a financial problem, it was that the Service was spending too little rather than too much. This applied particularly to capital expenditure, which averaged out at less than £10 million a year in the first years of the NHS. The Guillebaud Committee advocated an annual rate of hospital capital expenditure of £30 million, while an American observer writing in 1958 spoke for many when he commented: 'It is high time . . . to let the Health Service go on a spending spree, instead of continuing to subject it to the miserly penny-pinching necessary in the immediate post-war period.'[36]

A year later the *British Medical Journal* published a 'Report on Hospital Building', prepared by two consultant surgeons, Lawrence Abel and Walpole Lewin, at the invitation of the BMA.[37] The Report suggested that £750 million needed to be spent over a 10 year period on hospital building. The pressure to respond to these demands was clearly strong, and the appointment of Enoch Powell as Minister of Health in 1960 provided the political leadership required to establish a central government commitment to an expanding building programme. At Powell's instigation, regional hospital boards prepared development plans which were published in 1962 in The Hospital Plan. This envisaged a total expenditure of £500 million in the 10 years up to 1971, with building centring on a network of district general hospitals. The Hospital Plan was a major turning point in the evolution of the NHS as it marked the end of the era of 'make do and mend'. Although the Plan's proposals were soon found to be overambitious, and were revised in the 1966 Hospital Building Programme, they provided a framework of development for the next decade and beyond.

On the occasion of the publication of the Hospital Plan, the Ministry of Health invited local authorities to prepare ten year plans for the development of their health and welfare services. These plans were published in April 1963 as *Health and Welfare: the Development of Community Care*. This was essentially 'a collation of the relatively independent predictions, intentions or ambitions of departments in

146 individual authorities',[38] rather than a national programme of developments like the Hospital Plan.

It was nevertheless useful in providing information on local authorities' aspirations, particularly insofar as groups like the mentally ill, the mentally handicapped and the elderly were concerned, for whom care in the community was especially important. A revised version of the Health and Welfare Plan was published in 1966. Six years later the social services departments created as a result of the Seebohm reorganisation prepared ten year development plans. Like their predecessors, these were overambitious and were unevenly implemented. Nevertheless, all three planning exercises performed a function in that they encouraged a more systematic examination of service provision and enabled comparisons to be made between authorities.

Services for the mentally ill were subject to the greatest degree of change in the early 1960s. A decade earlier, in 1954, the mental hospital population had reached a peak, and thereafter declined, largely as the result of the use of new drugs. The Royal Commission on Mental Illness and Mental Deficiency which reported in 1957 recommended that the legal position with regard to mental disorder be liberalised, and this was done in the 1959 Mental Health Act. Thereafter almost all patients were treated on a voluntary basis, and the virtual elimination of locked wards became known as the 'open door' policy. Moreover, the Ministry of Health asked regional hospital boards to plan their services on the basis that only half the beds available for mental illness in 1960 would be needed in 1975. The Ministry had arrived at this target by using some questionable statistical evidence, leading critics to argue that the policy was inspired by a desire to save money rather than benefit patients. Whatever the reasons, the target was almost met, although for many patients the open door became the revolving door.

Somewhat paradoxically, while the early 1960s saw a number of major advances in the NHS, some commentators began to question the whole concept of a national health service. The most cogent critique came from Dennis Lees, who argued that medical care was no different from other consumer goods and so, like those goods, should be bought and sold by the market mechanism.[39] Lees advocated a system of private insurance for medical care in which political decisions about health services would be replaced by consumer choice. In a less fundamental way the NHS was also challenged by the new wave of patients' pressure groups which came into existence in the 1960s. The establishment of organisations like the National Association for the Welfare of Children in Hospital and the Patients' Association indicated growing discontent with the managers of the Service, and suggested that hospital boards and management committees had failed in their duty to represent patients. These groups, in actively asserting patients' rights and interests, also threatened the traditional dominance of the medical profession in the doctor-patient relationship.

A third challenge to the NHS, and in the long term the most influential, came in the form of the report of the Medical Services Review Committee, published in 1962. This Committee, under the chairmanship of Sir Arthur Porritt, had been set up by organisations representing the medical profession in 1958, and its members were chosen so that 'the status of the Committee should be such as to command the respect and confidence of the entire profession'.[40] Its terms of reference were to review the first 10 years' experience of the NHS and make recommendations for future development. In a wide-ranging report, the Committee reached two conclusions of particular importance. First, it affirmed its belief that 'the concept of a comprehensive national health service is sound'.[41] Given the profession's prevarications at the time of the establishment of the NHS, this was a statement of some significance. Second, the Committee concluded that the tripartite structure of the NHS was so 'fundamentally unsound' that 'no amount of touching up or improvisation can correct this basic defect in the Service'.[42] Accordingly, the establishment of area health boards was recommended, to be responsible for the planning and administration of all medical and ancillary services.

These views mirrored very closely the ideas outlined in the green paper, *The Administrative Structure of Medical and Related Services in England and Wales*, published in July 1968. This launched the debate about NHS reorganisation by suggesting that the tripartite structure needed to be replaced by a unified form of administration. A system in which 40 to 50 area boards might replace the multiplicity of authorities providing medical and related services, including regional hospital boards, was put forward for discussion. The issue of local government control of the new area boards was raised, but a decision was in part dependent on the unresolved question of the future structure of local government which was being debated at the same time. The green paper was critical of regional hospital boards, claiming that

> the interest which Regional Hospital Boards have increasingly taken in the performance of management functions by Hospital Management Committees, though not outside their statutory powers, may go beyond what was envisaged when the structure was established. Their primary task as originally conceived was planning and coordinating development; their intervention in matters of management has grown out of their responsibility for allocating financial resources, but is sometimes unwelcome. Confused responsibilities tend to create unsatisfactory relationships.[43]

Hence the proposal that there should be a direct relationship between the area boards and the central department.

Meanwhile, the training of doctors to staff the health service of the future continued and even expanded. Following the miscalculations of the Willink Committee, which in 1957 recommended that the intake to medical schools should be reduced, the number of medical students in training increased from the early 1960s, and received a further boost from the work of the Royal Commission on Medical Education, which reported in 1968. New medical schools were set up in Leicester, Nottingham and Southampton, and existing schools were expanded. However, dissatisfaction among established doctors came to the fore in 1966, when general practitioners negotiated a Doctors' Charter with the Ministry which led to a better deal for family doctors, and encouraged doctors to work from health centres. The development of health centres had been emphasised by Aneurin Bevan as one of the positive advantages to be gained from a national health service, but shortage of money and the lack of incentive to GPs meant that they were slow in getting off the ground. After 1966 they developed much faster. In the hospital service the main problem concerned the frustrations of junior doctors (those below consultant grade) with their terms and conditions of service and career prospects. This frustration was reflected also in the formation of the Junior Hospital Doctors' Association in 1966. Despite lengthy negotiations between the profession and the Ministry, and the establishment of new manpower planning machinery, the problems of hospital doctors continued into the 1970s.

The debate on NHS reorganisation started by the Porritt Report and the 1968 green paper identified lack of co-ordination between the different branches of the Service as one of the main deficiencies of the tripartite structure. This view was underlined by a series of reports from committees of enquiry investigating conditions in long-stay hospitals, starting with the Ely Report in 1969.[44] These reports were a reminder that, whatever the achievements of the NHS in other spheres, in the case of long-stay services much remained to be done. The Secretary of State for Social Services at the time of Ely, Richard Crossman, used the Report to give greater priority to these services. His two most significant initiatives were setting up the Hospital Advisory Service to visit and report on conditions at hospitals for the mentally ill, the mentally handicapped and the elderly; and the earmarking of money to be spent on these groups of patients.

It was also under Crossman that a new means of allocating money to regional hospital boards was devised. Traditionally, funds had been distributed on the basis of last year's allocation plus an addition to meet the cost of running new buildings (known as the revenue consequences of capital schemes) and other developments. This had succeeded in perpetuating the inequalities which existed in 1948, leaving London and the home counties far better off in terms of *per capita* expenditure than the rest of the country. A formula was worked out under Crossman, designed to reduce these inequalities over time, and it was introduced in 1971. A revised method of allocation was later worked out by the Resource Allocation Working Party (RAWP).

The rising cost of the NHS in the 1960s was another element in the reorganisation debate. Expenditure increased rapidly throughout this period, rising from £433 million in 1949 to £861 million in 1960 and £3000 million in 1973. It was not surprising then that a number of reports published in the mid 1960s should be concerned with the effectiveness of management in the hospital service, which accounted for two-thirds of the NHS budget. Of particular note were the Farquharson-Lang report on the administrative practices of Scottish hospital boards, the Cogwheel reports on the organisation of medical work, and the Salmon report on the nurse staffing structure.[45] The message from all three was that more effective management structures were required.

This message was taken to heart by the Ministry of Health, which in November 1968 was merged with the Ministry of Social Security to form the Department of Health and Social Security (DHSS). With assistance from the management consultants, McKinsey's, the new Department reviewed its own organisation, and by the end of 1972 had introduced a revised headquarters structure. The two most important effects for the NHS were the strengthening of the Department's links with field authorities through the establishment of new regional liaison and regional planning divisions; and the introduction of service development divisions based on patient groups, like the socially handicapped and children, in place of the policy divisions based solely on type of service – for example, the hospital service division.

As far as NHS reorganisation was concerned, a second green paper, *The Future Structure of the National Health Service*, was published in 1970.[46] This announced that a firm decision had been taken not to place the health service under the control of local government. Opposition from the medical profession and uncertainties about how to finance a health service run by local government appeared to be the main factors behind this decision. The proposals put forward in the first green paper were also unacceptable, because of the remoteness of the area boards from the people they served; the fear that boards might be hospital dominated; and the absence of a regional planning tier. To meet these criticisms the second green paper proposed the establishment of 90 area boards, together with 14 regional health councils with advisory and planning functions, and 200 district committees as a channel of local participation.

The change of government in 1970 led to a third set of proposals in the form of the Consultative Document, circulated to interested organisations in May 1971. The Consultative Document was in some respects an extension of the two green papers. Thus it accepted the arguments for a unified system of administration in the shape of regional and area health authorities. Local participation was catered for by the proposal that community health councils should be set up to express the views of the public to health authorities. The Document differed from the green papers in the greater emphasis it placed on effective management. It proposed that the administrative structure should be based on the principle of 'maximum delegation downwards, matched by accountability upwards',[47] and that there should be a clear definition of responsibilities for each tier of authority. Also, health authorities would have a small membership –

around fifteen members each including a chairman – and 'management ability will be the main criterion for the selection of members'.[48] Again, an 'expert study' of the detailed management arrangements of the new authorities would be carried out.[49] The Consultative Document continued the trend set by the green papers by further strengthening the powers of the regional tier. Finally, it was announced that the boundaries of area health authorities would match those of local authorities, and a working party was established to look at collaboration between the NHS and local government.[50] These proposals were later amplified in the white paper, *National Health Service Reorganisation in England*, published in August 1972,[51] and formed the basis of the NHS Act 1973. After six years of debate the NHS was reorganised on 1 April 1974.

This synoptic overview has pointed to the main trends and milestones in the NHS in its first phase. The picture painted has necessarily been both general and national, and no more than a broad-brush coverage has been attempted. The more subtle shades and finer details will be added in the following chapters, beginning with an examination of the way in which the Leeds Regional Hospital Board organised its work.

2

The Organisation of the Board's Work

This chapter explains how the Leeds Regional Hospital Board went about organising its work. The chapter begins with a brief description of the Leeds Region, and then discusses how Board members were appointed. Particular attention is given to the turnover of members and their role. This is followed by an account of the relationship between the Board's officers. The next section examines the Board's committee system and the respective role of members and officers. Then an account is given of the way in which hospitals in the Region were organised into groups run by hospital management committees. Finally, the Board's reaction to the debate on health service reorganisation is discussed. Overall, the chapter provides a context for the more detailed analyses which follow. It also contains data relevant to a number of issues of recurring interest in the NHS, including consensus management, the role of members, and the nature and pace of administrative change.

The Leeds Region

Shortly after the 1946 National Health Service Act had been passed the Ministry of Health issued regulations defining the areas of the hospital regions. The Act had specified that 'the Minister shall secure, so far as practicable, that each area is such that the provision of the said services in the area can conveniently be associated with a university having a school of medicine', and Aneurin Bevan had spoken of 16 to 20 such areas being formed. In the event, he decided on 14, and the Leeds Region, which was to be associated with the medical school at the University of Leeds, was defined as:

The administrative counties of the East Riding of York, the North Riding of York (except the part included in the Newcastle Regional Hospital Area) and the West Riding of York (except the part included in the Sheffield Regional Hospital Area). The county boroughs of Bradford, Dewsbury, Halifax, Huddersfield, Kingston-upon-Hull, Leeds, Wakefield and York.

As thus defined, the Region covered 4237 square miles and contained some three million people. The bulk of this population was concentrated in the manufacturing towns of the centre and south, where the woollen and ready-made clothing trades, and, to a lesser extent, coal mining, were the major sources of employment. Hull, the only sizable town in the east, was dominated by the shipping, fishing and the coastal trades, and was noted for its insularity. These urban areas contrasted strongly with the dales in the north-west and the plain which extended from York to the coast, where the scattered populace was engaged mainly in agriculture and related activities.[1] The main features of the Region are indicated in Figure 2.1.

Once the areas of the hospital regions had been decided, the next step was the appointment of board members. The Act had stipulated that, before making these appointments, the Minister should consult local health authorities, organisations representing the medical profession, associated universities, and any other bodies which appeared to be concerned. In making the first appointments, Bevan and his advisers included voluntary hospitals in the last category. The membership of all 14 boards was announced in July 1947 and, of the 24 members of the Leeds Board, 7 came from local authorities, 6 from voluntary hospitals, and 10 from professions in the medical field, including 4 university professors, 4 consultants, one general practitioner, and a matron. The membership was completed by a trade unionist. John E. Fattorini, who was chairman of the Bradford Royal Infirmary, was named as the Board's first chairman. The Minister was at pains to stress that while the boards' members might be connected with various organisations, these organisations had no right of nomination and members were neither representatives nor delegates of their parent bodies, but had been chosen for the contribution they could make as individuals. He hoped that members would sacrifice their existing loyalties to the good of the hospital service as a whole and, to this end, as well as striving for a mix of medical, lay, municipal and voluntary hospital members, Bevan

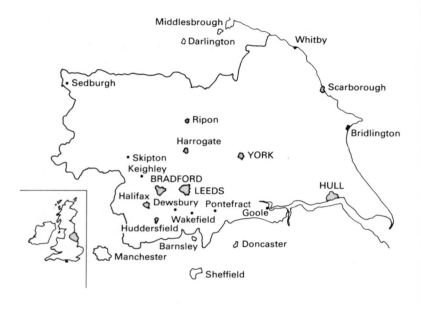

FIGURE 2.1   Area covered by the Leeds Regional Hospital Board

sought to distribute membership reasonably over each region on a territorial basis.

At the outset, one-third of the members successively came up for reappointment in the years 1949, 1950 and 1951. After these initial arrangements, the term of office became three years and no upper limit was placed on the number of times a person could be reappointed. Boards themselves were consulted when vacancies arose or when reappointments were necessary, and in the latter case the Leeds Board invariably recommended the reappointment *en bloc* of retiring members.

This was what led a later Secretary of State for Social Services, Richard Crossman, to describe boards as 'self-perpetuating oligar-chies'.[2] It was, however, entirely up to the Minister to decide whether to accept the advice given, and in a number of cases new people were appointed. Thus, in the period up to 31 March 1953, 37 people were members of the Leeds Board, representing a turnover of 50 per cent in just under six years. A total of 82 people sat on the Board during the course of its life, and only one of these was a member throughout the whole period. Again, the Board was served by four chairmen: on his death in 1949, Fattorini was succeeded by Alderman H. Bambridge, who in turn was succeeded by Major J. C. Hunter in 1955. Both Bambridge and Hunter had served as vice-chairmen, but this was not true of L. E. Laycock, who became chairman in 1963: indeed, Laycock had not even been a member of the Board. But the important point to note is that the turnover of members and chairmen suggests that boards were not as self-perpetuating as Crossman maintained.

What was the role of members? Local government control of the NHS having been rejected, it seems that boards of appointed members were included in the administrative structure of the Service for two reasons: first, to subject the work of full-time officers to some kind of public control and scrutiny; and, secondly, to introduce an element of community representation. In theory, then, members combined a management role with a representative role, but in practice the situation was a good deal more complicated. On the basis of interviews and documentary evidence, it has been possible to identify six roles which members played on the Leeds Board. The first was to represent local interests. Board members were drawn from different areas within the Region, and some came to see their principal function as being to defend and promote the interests of those areas. In the eyes of those interviewed, Hull members were particularly inclined to be parochial, and the geographical isolation of the city, together with poor road and rail links, may account for this. Secondly, there was the special interest role. Some members, by virtue of their experience and group membership, had a special knowledge of certain areas of service provision, like mental health. They were active on the appropriate committees of the Board, and became known as the spokesmen for these services. Thirdly, and very much connected with this, there was the role of patients' representative, mainfested in the visits to hospitals, particularly long-stay hospitals, undertaken by members as a means of keeping a check on standards of care and patient welfare. Fourthly, there was the professional interest role, seen most clearly in the medical membership of the Board, which amounted to one-quarter of total membership. Fifthly, there was the role of looking after, or at least speaking up for, the interests of other organisations, such as local authorities and the board of governors of the Leeds teaching hospital. Finally, there was the role of manager of services and allocator of resources. This tended to be concentrated in the chairman and a small number of other senior members, whose principal concern was the most effective and efficient use of resources.

These roles have been separated here for analytical purposes, whereas in fact there was considerable overlap. What they demonstrate is that in practice it was difficult for members to follow the Ministry's advice and ignore their existing loyalties. This is not to say that Board meetings were always occasions when different interests confronted one another: far from it. But roles were shaped, inevitably, by members' commitments to other organisations and interests, and Board meetings were a stage where these roles were played out. This, however, is to see only half the picture, for we must also examine the role of officers in the Board's work.

The officers of the Board

The Leeds Board met for the first time on 3 July 1947 and it immediately decided to advertise the posts of its two principal officers,[3] the Senior Administrative Medical Officer (SAMO) and Secretary. Candidates for the former were required to be 'registered medical practitioners with wide general and hospital administrative experience', and a salary of £2250 was offered; candidates for the latter were required to have 'wide administrative experience and will be responsible for the Board's business management, including general supervision of the Finance, Supply and Establishment organisation', and in this case the salary was £1400. Interviews for these posts were held in September, and as a result Dr A. B. Williamson was appointed as SAMO and W. A. Shee as Secretary. Both men came from local government backgrounds – Williamson having been Medical Officer of Health of the City of Portsmouth, and Shee, County Public Assistance Officer in Gloucestershire. That Williamson and Shee came from outside the Region was not without significance, since interests within the Region had been pressing their own favourites for appointment. But a majority of members felt it was desirable to select as officers men without existing loyalties, and so it was that the appointments were made. Williamson and Shee took up their duties on 1st November 1947. At the same time steps were taken to fill the two chief officer posts, and a Treasurer was appointed at the end of 1947, followed by an Architect early in 1948. A Nursing Officer was added to the chief officer establishment in 1950. The core of officers remained the same until 1961, when, as a result of the expanding building programme, a Regional Engineer was appointed. Otherwise the main feature worth noting on the staffing side is the appointment of a number of specialist administrative staff just below chief officer level: a Regional Catering Adviser in 1956, a Regional Supplies Officer in 1969, a Regional Information Officer in 1970, and a Regional Pharmacist in 1972.

The influence exerted by officers on the Board's work was one of the points stressed repeatedly by those interviewed during the research, and particular mention was made of the troubled relationship between the first Secretary and SAMO. At least part of the problem was that the relative status of SAMOs and Secretaries was never precisely defined by the Ministry of Health. (There is a nice contrast here with the detailed role specifications handed down in the Grey Book at the time of NHS reorganisation.[4]) From the difference in salaries, however, it might be deduced that the SAMO was the senior of the two. This would be supported by the need for the SAMO to be university educated, a qualification not required of the Secretary. Yet the SAMO's seniority was not specified by the Ministry, which seemed to take the view that the two officers were co-equals and that the relationship was best left to work itself out in practice. This meant that much would depend on the personalities involved. It seemed natural that responsibility for advising the Board on all medical administrative matters would rest with the SAMO, while the Secretary would be pre-eminent on matters of general administration. This left a no-man's-land in between, open to dispute. How this would be resolved clearly depended on the spirit in which the SAMO and Secretary worked together.

Matters were not helped in the Leeds Region by the completely different personalities of the SAMO and Secretary. Consequently, relationships between the medical and lay administrative sides of the Board were not always harmonious, particularly at the most senior level. This was mentioned frequently during interviews, and there is also documentary evidence of the disagreements and conflicts which occurred between the two men. For example, in 1954 the Board, at the request of the SAMO, formed a special committee of its most senior members to 'clarify and define the question of seniority and the relative duties and responsibilities of its Chief Officers'. The committee met on five occasions and, as well as examining relevant documentary evidence, it sought the Ministry's advice. In reporting to the Board the committee recommended no change in the respective duties and responsibilities of the SAMO and Secretary, adding that it had

> made known to the officers its opinion that, as regards social functions, invitations from outside bodies were entirely matters for those bodies concerned and there should be no interference; and that, as to official occasions sponsored by the Board, the members looked to the two officers themselves to decide any question of status or precedence, having regard to the nature of the occasion, and that, in the event of a disagreement, it should be a matter for the Chairman to decide.

The Committee concluded that it believed

> That its meetings have assisted materially to clear away misunderstandings that existed, and further, that, if the decisions contained in this report are accepted without reservation by all concerned, difficulties which have arisen in the past will no longer arise, and it is hoped that the result will be a happier relationship between all concerned.

Unfortunately this did not happen, and there was a further disagreement in 1957 when a request from the SAMO that certain members of the administrative and clerical staff employed in the medical section of the Board should be upgraded was turned down by the Secretary. Another special committee was appointed, and the Board again took the Ministry's advice. When the matter came before the Staff and Establishment Committee members took the unusual step of excluding the officers, and when the latter were recalled they were informed that 'in order to clarify any doubts, the Senior Administrative Medical Officer was regarded as the Board's chief adviser in medical matters, and that the Secretary was the chief administrative officer in all matters affecting the general administration of the Board'. Commenting on precisely this issue some ten years later, the Farquharson-Lang Committee found that: 'There was general agreement among our witnesses that it was very difficult to determine the dividing line between 'medical' and 'non-medical' administration . . . and that this could sometimes give rise to difficulty, both for the boards and officers concerned.[5] This certainly applied to the Leeds Region.

These examples serve to illustrate the continuing struggle for power and precedence between the SAMO and Secretary. It is also worth noting that relationships between the Secretary and Treasurer and the Secretary and Architect were sometimes uneasy. Thus the 1954 investigation of chief officers' duties and responsibilities, referred to above, was in part a response to the Treasurer's concern at the Secretary's close supervision and involvement in his work, which the Treasurer had brought to the attention of the Board's Chairman as early as 1949. Again, in the early 1950s the Secretary had taken steps to tighten up on procedures in the Architect's department, thereby causing some friction.

The main struggle, though, was between the SAMO and Secretary, and, in a general review of the relationship between Secretaries and SAMOs conducted in 1957, the Action Society postulated four courses which might be followed: the Secretary could be declared the senior; the SAMO could be declared the senior; the Chairman could take control; or the relationship could be left to work itself out in practice.[6] The documentary sources do not reveal which of these courses was followed in the Leeds Region, but, in the opinion of almost all of those interviewed during the research, while Fattorini was Chairman he was leader of the Board and held sway over the officers. There was a strong feeling among the interviewees that after Fattorini's death in 1949 the Secretary asserted his pre-eminence and gradually increased his control over the Board's work. At the same time, the SAMO continued to press the claims of medical administration, and to resist any attempts by the Secretary to intervene in medical matters. One of the consequences was the development of disagreements of the kind noted above, in which the Board itself was called in to adjudicate.

Later changes in personnel showed that conflict did not necessarily inhere in the nature of the posts. Dr Williamson retired in 1959 and was succeeded by Dr A. A. Driver, who had previously been deputy SAMO in the Liverpool Region, and assistant SAMO in the Leeds Region. Also at the beginning of his career he had worked at St James's Hospital, Leeds, and so he had considerable knowledge of hospital services in the Region. Shee retired in 1963 and was succeeded as Secretary by W. Bowring, who had previously been group secretary to the Wakefield (B) HMC and before that group secretary to the Pontefract and Castleford HMC. Earlier still, Bowring had been on the Board's staff, as Assistant Secretary between 1948 and 1950, and so like Driver he brought much experience to his new responsibilities.

According to those interviewed, the relationship between Driver and Bowring was much more harmonious than that between Williamson and Shee. The two men had a mutual respect for each other's abilities and spheres of concern, and worked as the co-equals which the Ministry had envisaged. On the other hand, during the period when Shee and Driver were in office together, most of the interviewees argued that Shee continued to dominate the Board's work. This is supported by documentary evidence, such as that on the building of a new hospital at Eastburn, which is worth considering in a little detail.

The origins of the Eastburn scheme go back to an appraisal of the development of St Luke's Hospital, Huddersfield, prepared in November 1962. The St Luke's project had been designed by the architects, Poulsons, in a very short time, and had been standardised as far as possible. The result was a much lower cost than in comparable schemes. Encouraged by this, Shee raised with the Ministry of Health the possibility of applying similar principles to the building of a complete general hospital. In February 1963 he was asked to explore this possibility, and Poulsons were commissioned to prepare a plan for what became known as 'P.G.H. 600', to denote a peripheral general hospital of 600 beds.

The plan was received from Poulsons just 27 days later, and it was forwarded to the Ministry early in April 1963. The plan suggested that a 600 bed peripheral general hospital could be built at a cost of £4000 a bed, on the principles used in the Huddersfield scheme. The Ministry responded enthusiastically, and towards the end of May 1963 the Board was invited to submit a proposal for the building of such a hospital. At very short notice, Board members were called to an informal discussion and agreed in principle to accept the Ministry's invitation.

The enthusiasm of the Ministry's response caught the Board's members and medical staff somewhat unawares. This much is clear from the detailed note of a General Purposes Committee Meeting of 13 June 1963, which was the first formal opportunity for Board members to discuss the scheme. The SAMO, Dr A. A. Driver, told members that: 'It was a tribute to Mr Shee's advocacy that the Ministry had seen fit to commit itself so quickly'.

The significance of the 'P.G.H. 600' project in the context of the hospital building programme is discussed in Chapter 3. The point to note here is the way in which Shee took up the issue and persuaded the Ministry to support his initiative. Of particular relevance to the present argument is the development of the project in its initial stages with little reference to the views of the SAMO and his colleagues.

To summarise, then, relationships between the Board's officers have been discussed at some length because of the importance of these relationships for those interviewed during the research, and because of the more general lessons for management in the NHS. Perhaps the most obvious lesson is that, in a situation where principal officers are given equal status and are enjoined to work together, the personalities involved become important. Later attempts to achieve consensus management, and particularly failures in such attempts, point to a similar conclusion.[7]

Establishing the Organisation

It was a number of years before the Board settled on an established organisational routine. Permanent office accommodation was not found until March 1951, and so before that date the monthly meetings of the Board were held in hospitals throughout the Region. A novel feature of the Board's work in these early years was the holding of policy meetings separately from ordinary monthly meetings. On three occasions – in September 1949, October 1950 and May 1952 – members of the Board, together with the principal and chief officers, met for three days in succession to review the development of hospital and specialist services in the Region and to decide future policy. The officers prepared background briefing papers and the chairmen of the standing committees reported on progress in their spheres, the idea being that members should rise above the concern with details which characterised ordinary monthly meetings and look at long-term strategic policy issues. Most members felt that this aim was achieved. The reason why policy meetings were discontinued after 1952 was that by then the Board had so organised its work that it was no longer necessary to hold special meetings for this purpose.

Evidence of this greater degree of organisation in the Board's work was the adoption of standing orders in March 1950. As well as laying down rules for the conduct of meetings, these set out in detail the size and functions of committees. By this time there were 11 standing committees, of which the most important was the General Purposes Committee which comprised the whole of the members of the Board. In addition, there were three advisory committees, numerous special committees which were formed at various times to deal with particular matters, and a number of liaison committees. Procedure was refined further in 1952 when it was agreed that Board meetings should be held in alternate months instead of monthly. The same principle was applied to committees, with the major standing committees meeting in the months when the Board did not, thus facilitating the flow of minutes between the two.

This method and form of organisation was not seriously questioned until 1967, when the Ministry of Health asked boards to give careful consideration to the recommendations of the Farquharson-Lang Committee. This Committee had looked at the role of hospital board members and officers in Scotland, but its findings were of wider applicability. Drawing an analogy with industry, the Committee argued that members were comparable to a board of directors. This implied that the chairman should not become the managing director but should leave this task to the officers. Moreover, since the chairman and members could not be expected to give much more than 12 hours a month to board work, they should concentrate on formulating broad policy, deciding priorities, setting objectives and checking to see whether these objectives had been met. The execution of policy and day-to-day management would thus be delegated to officers. Further, if board members were to concentrate their attention on wider issues, then the number of committees employed by boards would have to be reduced as these committees took up a great deal of members' time. In sum, the Committee suggested that there was a 'need for a general reappraisal by all boards of the respective functions of members and officers, to ensure that the best use is made of the particular talents and skills of each category'.[8]

After considering the Committee's report the Leeds Board made two changes in its own arrangements. First, the Board decided to reduce the number of standing committees by one by amalgamating the Finance Committee and General Purposes Committee. Secondly, responsibility for certain minor matters like attendances of non-medical staff at courses and conferences was delegated to the officers.

Clearly, these were token gestures which did little to change the established practices of the Board.

Nevertheless, the Farquharson-Lang Committee did raise important questions about the role of members and the relationship between members and officers. In the Leeds Region members did become heavily involved in management issues through the extensive network of committees that had been set up. Their knowledge of services was in many cases substantial, and was used to justify a close involvement in policy making. Whether this resulted in the neglect of broader priority-setting and monitoring functions and responsibilities is difficult to judge from the available documentary evidence. The decision to discontinue special policy meetings would suggest not, and members certainly did debate major developments like the Hospital Plan: not only this, but members also contributed to the detailed proposals which went into the Plan, as is shown in the next chapter. What does emerge is that of the six member roles outlined earlier in this chapter, the role of patients' representative was the least well articulated. The interests of localities, particular services, professional groups and local authorities are not always the same as those of patients, and it was the former which tended to predominate. Also, the management role of members was emphasised, particularly by the Farquharson-Lang Committee, which dealt almost exclusively with the management functions of boards, making only passing reference to their work as 'consumer councils'.[9] Perhaps one of the reasons why the patients' representative role was not well articulated at Regional Board level was that it was seen to be more a function of hospital management committees.

As far as the relationship between members and officers was concerned, there was a general feeling among those interviewed that the Board's first Secretary, W. A. Shee, had a commanding influence over the Board's work, and that he tended to dominate the members and chairman, with the exception of Fattorini, in the same way that he tended to dominate the other officers. After Shee's retirement a more equal relationship developed between both officers, and officers and members. By virtue of being full-time officials and having command over information, the officers were undoubtedly in a strong position. In contrast, members had neither the support of a party machine nor the electoral power base of members of local authorities. This meant that the overall balance of power was tilted towards the officers. Yet their power was not total, and issues did arise where members took a lead in policy making. This was certainly true of services for the elderly and the mentally ill, which are discussed in Chapter 5. Another important point, hinted at earlier, is that the chairman and a small number of other senior members tended to work particularly closely with the officers on management and resource-allocation issues. Taking account of these qualifications, the decision-making system at Board level is perhaps best described as pluralistic, with different interests winning out over different issues. It is the interplay of these interests, and their impact on other interests outside the Board, which forms the subject of the following chapters.

Hospital Management Committees

With characteristic understatement, the Ministry of Health made the following observation on the setting up of the NHS:

> Though the patient who went to sleep in a hospital bed on the evening of the 4th July probably did not notice anything very different when he woke up on the morning of the 5th, the administrative complications of the transfer were considerable.[10]

One of these complications was the need to establish hospital management committees (HMCs) to take over responsibility for hospitals from local authorities and voluntary hospital boards. This was an issue which took up a good deal of the time of the Leeds Board in the first nine months of its existence. The problem facing the Board could be stated simply: how to group 209 hospitals, 10 convalescent homes and 47 clinics, containing some 34 000 beds, into units which were manageable as regards day-to-day administration. After extensive discussions by members and officers with those responsible for the local management of hospitals, a scheme was devised for the creation of 22 groups of hospitals. The Ministry of Health responded favourably, but suggested that a separate group be formed to administer hospitals in the Goole area. This was accepted, with the result that 23 groups were established.

The number of hospitals in these groups ranged from 18 in the Dewsbury area to what was effectively a single hospital in the case of Storthes Hall, a mental illness hospital near Huddersfield. The variation in bed complements was just as great, rising from a minimum of 400 in the Goole area to around 3000 in those groups which included a large mental illness hospital. One of the most interesting aspects of the scheme lay in the treatment of mental hospitals, where the Board experimented by creating groups with a mental hospital only, a large mental hospital combined with a general hospital, and a mental hospital combined with a group of general hospitals. Only the Leeds and Birmingham Regions adopted this approach;[11] elsewhere, a policy of almost complete separation was pursued. It is not clear which system of administration was most beneficial to mental-illness hospitals, although Jones has argued that mental-handicap hospitals suffered from being included in groups with general hospitals.[12]

Each hospital group was administered by a HMC whose members were appointed by the Board. In making these appointments the Board consulted various interests, and it decided to allocate membership according to the following rough guide: 25 per cent to be appointed after consultation with local authorities; 25 per cent after consultation with the governing bodies of voluntary hospitals; 20 per cent after consultation with senior hospital medical and dental staff; 15 per cent after consultation with executive councils; and 15 per cent after consultation with other interested organisations – such as the Yorkshire Trades Council, the British Medical Association, the County Federation of Women's Institutes, and local medical committees. The interests consulted remained the same throughout the period 1948–74, except that voluntary associations replaced the governing bodies of voluntary hospitals after the initial series of appointments.

The membership of HMCs in the Leeds Region ranged from 16 to 28. In addition, each committee had a specially selected chairman. Despite the Ministry's advice that a *limited* degree of dual membership was desirable, but only 'very exceptionally' should Board members be HMC chairmen, 7 of the 23 chairmen sat on the Board, and a further 8 Board members were also HMC members, some of these even being appointed to serve on more than one committee. Later research revealed that this was common practice in other Regions.[13] The Board members who were interviewed argued that the closer contacts and local knowledge which resulted from overlapping membership helped further good relations between the Board and HMCs.

The original groupings remained the same until 1964, although in 1952 the Board had unsuccessfully approached the Ministry of

Health with a proposal to enlarge certain groups by amalgamation. The Ministry's advice had been that small groups were preferable, but policy had changed by 1964 when the group that had been created specially to administer two sanatoria in the north-west of the Region was amalgamated with an adjacent group. Two years later the hospitals in the small Goole group were transferred to the control of other HMCs. These moves were given added impetus by the Farquharson-Lang Report, and further amalgamations reduced the number of hospital groups in the Region to 18. Also, the number of members on management committees was reduced, in line with the Report's argument that if membership became too large 'this will tend to defeat the [management committee's] broad management function and to convert it into a body which can only endorse the activities of its committees and exercise a very limited co-ordinating function'.[14] Membership of HMCs was cut from around 500 in 1967 to some 300 in 1973 and, whereas all HMCs had over 20 members in 1967, the maximum number advocated by the Ministry, by 1973 no HMC had more than this number. At the same time, management committees were streamlining their own procedures, for example by delegating more responsibility to officers and cutting down on the number of sub-committees used. These evolutionary reforms were, however, soon overtaken by the more fundamental reorganisation of the NHS in 1974.

Reorganisation

The national developments leading up to NHS reorganisation have been described in the previous chapter. It will come as no surprise to discover that the Leeds Board's reaction to the various proposals that were put forward became more favourable as the reorganisation debate proceeded, particularly as greater emphasis came to be placed on some form of regional organisation. Klein has argued that the reinstatement of the regional tier may reflect 'a sort of political law of gravity which states that, in the absence of countervailing pulls, everything will tend to return to the point of departure'.[15] Whatever the explanation, the final form of reorganisation met with the approval of the Board.

While reorganisation had several aims, a factor stressed by the 1970–4 Conservative Government which piloted through the necessary legislation was the need for more effective management. This was consistent with the philosophy behind a number of health service developments in the late 1960s and early 1970s, including the Farquharson-Lang Report, the Salmon Report on the nurse staffing structure, and the Cogwheel Reports on the organisation of medical work. At a more prosaic level, the search for greater management efficiency was seen in the growth of the Board's Organisation and Methods and Work Study Unit, which increased in size from 9 staff in 1966 to 30 seven years later.

Brown has argued that this emphasis on better management was a reflection of the 1960s climate of opinion that the main problems facing public services were of a technical nature amenable to administrative solutions.[16] NHS reorganisation and the simultaneous reform of local government were the highest expression of this. Yet the question remains as to whether wholesale restructuring of the kind experienced in 1974 was to be preferred to more incremental changes. Brown's work has demonstrated that fundamental reform carries its own costs which are often not included in the calculus of change. If, as seems likely, Brown's conclusions are more widely applicable, then less drastic changes, based on local needs rather than a national blueprint, may represent a better way forward.

This was precisely the approach advocated by the Leeds Board in response to the first green paper. The Board maintained that 'an evolutionary rather than a revolutionary course would be preferable and consideration should be given as to where and how the existing Service could be improved'. The policy of rationalising the HMC structure was one area in which the Board felt that this policy could be pursued. Other suggestions included placing teaching hospitals, ambulance services and executive council services under the control of a regional authority, which by implication would be a revamped regional hospital board. The prime need, though, was to proceed gradually, and not to promulgate radical reform.

These views were not, of course, accepted, although in retrospect some commentators felt that evolutionary change would have been better. What happened in practice was that on 1 April 1974 the Leeds Board and the 18 HMCs in the Region were superseded by the Yorkshire Regional Health Authority and seven area health authorities. The new Region was slightly larger than the old, and the functions of the new authorities were expanded to include responsibility for teaching hospitals and community health services and closer connections with family practitioner and local authority services.

At the final meeting of the Board, held on the 14 March 1974, the chairman, Sir Leslie Laycock, listed some of the achievements of the hospital service in the Region, and it is appropriate to conclude this chapter by reiterating some of the points made by Laycock. The number of new out-patients seen in the Region's hospitals had risen from 260 000 in 1949 to 386 000 in 1973, and total out-patient attendances had increased from 1 100 000 to 1 700 000. Over the same period discharges and deaths had increased from 177 000 to 330 000 a year and, as the number of beds available had fallen, turnover per bed had risen from 5.5 to 11.4. On the expenditure side, the Region's hospitals cost £89 million to run in 1973/1974 compared with just over £10 million in 1949/1950; and capital expenditure had increased from £435 000 in 1949/1950 to £10.87 million in 1973/1974, a total of £87 million having been spent over the 25 years.

These bare statistics are one way of summarising the Board's work. In the chapters which follow we shall examine other aspects of that work, and in so doing we hope to bring out the political and organisational complexities of decision making in the health service.

3

Planning

The wartime hospital surveys carried out by the Ministry of Health and the Nuffield Provincial Hospitals Trust had demonstrated a clear need for some kind of body to plan and co-ordinate the rather chaotic collection of services that existed in 1945. This was the principal *raison d'être* for regional hospital boards, whose main function was the planning of hospital and specialist services. Our purpose in this chapter is to describe how the Leeds Board went about this task. However, since descriptive data are of limited value, we also seek to analyse the Board's experience as a planning agency. In doing so we have been guided by the following questions, which it may be helpful to discuss briefly at the outset.

The first question we have asked about the Board's planning activities is: *Who was involved*? There are several possible participants, including officers and members of the Board and HMCs, officials from the Ministry of Health (and later DHSS), members of the medical profession, other agencies like local authorities, the public, and so on. A contrast can be drawn between highly participative systems on the one hand, and systems involving a small group of planners on the other. Secondly: *What approach to planning was used*? Writers on planning and decision theory have articulated a number of approaches ranging from the rational-comprehensive to incrementalism. In the rational-comprehensive model planners carry out a broad search of their policy world; identify goals and means of reaching those goals; evaluate the variety of options available; and then select the option whose consequences rank highest. In the incrementalist model policy-makers deal with problems as they arise, examine a small range of alternatives, and choose an alternative which represents only a small change from the *status quo*. Which approach best fits the Board's planning style? Thirdly, in the planning process: *How was the problem defined*? What deficiencies and shortcomings were identified by the participants? Fourthly: *What was the policy response*? Having defined a problem or group of problems, what proposals did the Board respond with? Of particular interest in the NHS context is how far the response entailed new building or other service developments; in other words, whether the emphasis was on capital planning or service planning. Fifthly: *How was this policy implemented*? Once a policy response had been agreed, what steps were taken to carry it out, and what obstacles were encountered? Sixthly: *Whose will prevailed*? Planning, like other forms of policy-making, often, though not always, involves a conflict between the various interests involved. When this happens, who wins and, when conflict does not occur, are some interests being suppressed? Finally: *Who benefited*? Planning involves taking decisions about the allocation of scarce resources, which means that some groups, interests, services and areas benefit and others do not. Is it possible to identify the winners (and losers) in health planning?

Rationalisation

'Rationality' and 'rationalisation' were two words which occurred frequently in discussions of hospital planning at the beginning of the NHS. They were usually compared – favourably – with disorganisation and duplication which were felt to characterise hospital services before 1948. Eckstein has captured the dominant philosophy of planning in the early years of the NHS in the following words:

> The purpose of planning, in a word, is to 'rationalise' the activities on which planning is imposed: to make subject to calculation what was previously left to chance, to organise what was previously unorganised, to replace spontaneous adjustments with deliberate control.[1]

How did the Leeds Board pursue these goals?

Lacking any information about hospital services in the Region apart from the wartime Hospital Survey, the Board called for its own survey to be carried out. This task was entrusted to the Board's medical advisory committees, which were composed mainly of consultants. On the basis of the knowledge of their own members, visits to hospitals, evidence from other doctors, and questionnaires completed by HMC secretaries, these committees built up a picture of services in each specialty. Then, by applying bed norms to each area, they identified those areas most in need of additional accommodation. The committees adopted their own bed norms in place of the Ministry of Health's recommended figures, which were rejected as unrealistically high.[2] The reports which resulted were considered in the first six months of 1949 by the Board's main medical advisory committee, the Specialist Services Advisory Committee, which comprised the medical members of the Board and two co-opted consultants. Following consultation with HMCs the Committee prepared a summary of services provided in each part of the Region. This was complemented by reports from the Senior Administrative Medical Officer (SAMO) and his assistants, who visited all hospitals in the Region before and during the first year of the NHS. These documents provided the main body of information on which the Board's initial planning decisions were made.

The first point to note, therefore, is that the principal participants in the planning process were drawn from the medical profession – that is, the Board's own medical members and officers – and senior doctors drafted on to advisory committees. The approach they used involved taking a general overview of services and then examining in more detail particular problem areas: an approach best described as 'mixed scanning', a term coined by Etzioni to describe behaviour somewhere between comprehensive rationality and incrementalism.[3] But what problems were thrown up by the survey?

The two main deficiencies identified were the overall shortage of beds throughout the Region, and inequalities in the distribution of beds between different areas. Thus both Huddersfield and Pontefract had serious bed shortages, but it was the Hull and East Riding area which was designated 'the most deficient in the Region for all needs and should, therefore, have priority attention'. At the opposite extreme was Halifax, which was described as 'one of the best areas in the Region from the point of view of the immediate availability of beds'. The survey went on to comment on the poor standard of much of the accommodation, which had suffered both war damage and wartime neglect. In the nine years up to 1948 there had been little new building, and maintenance expenditure had been reduced to a minimum because of more pressing demands on public expenditure and resources. The result was a backlog of work urgently needing to be carried out.

It was not surprising, then, that the Specialist Services Advisory Committee's main recommendation was that a heavy investment of capital expenditure was required. However, conscious that this would not be possible in the immediate post-war austerity years, the Committee suggested a number of ways in which the more obvious inadequacies could be ameliorated without great expense. These included: first, the reallocation of beds to specialties to distribute the overall shortage of accommodation more equally; secondly, the concentration in a single unit in each district hospital centre[4] of beds in specialties like ear, nose and throat (ENT), gynaecology and paediatrics, which were often scattered inefficiently among a number of small departments in several hospitals; thirdly, the co-ordination of infectious diseases hospitals in a regional scheme to release surplus beds for other uses; and, fourthly, the centralisation and extension of out-patient clinics to take pressure off in-patient waiting lists. The Board accepted the Committee's recommendations, and asked for further more detailed reports from its medical staff on how they might be implemented.

The report which followed on out-patient facilities showed that Hull and Huddersfield again had the highest priority for development, because waiting times for out-patient treatment were longest in those areas. Schemes for the improvement of out-patient facilities in Hull and Huddersfield were therefore put in hand, and facilities in other parts of the Region were also extended. As a consequence of the development of these facilities, there was a considerable increase in workload: between 1949 and 1955 the number of new out-patients seen in the Region's hospitals increased from 262 000 to 295 000, while total out-patient attendance rose from 1 114 000 to 1 164 000.

Over the same period the Board took action on another of the Specialist Services Advisory Committee's recommendations – the rationalisation of infectious diseases hospitals. Before 1948 many of the small fever hospitals were not used, and those that were did not work to full capacity. As the Hospital Survey commented: 'In no other section of hospital provision have the surveyors been so struck with the waste of buildings, equipment and skilled staff'.[5] On the advice of the SAMO, the Leeds Board decided to concentrate infectious diseases provision in 13 key hospitals, with 4 other hospitals being held in reserve for use in the events of epidemics. Of the remaining 34 hospitals, 12 were so unsuited to hospital purposes that there was no option but to dispose of them, while the other 22 became available for alternative uses, mainly for geriatric and chronic sick cases.

As the incidence of infectious diseases declined in later years, and as a higher proportion of the available beds were provided in cubicles, further reductions were effected. Indeed, one of the major changes in the first 25 years of the NHS was the fall in hospital provision for infectious diseases: in 1973 there were fewer than 400 infectious disease beds in the Region, compared with about 1800 in 1949, more than half of the reduction occurring between 1949 and 1953. The waste noted by the Hospital Survey was thus rapidly eliminated, and the benefits of regional planning were clearly visible.

These benefits proved more difficult to realise in the case of general hospital provision, although some progress was made. The initial allocations of beds to specialties in the Region were based on the recommendations of the Board's medical advisory committees and were intended to overcome the more obvious examples of duplication and shortages. In a report to the Board in October 1950 the SAMO stated that although these allocations had served their purpose for the planning of services in the early stages, they 'left much to be desired as an indication of the most effective permanent distribution of the available accommodation'. He argued that there was a need to ensure that 'patients in all parts of the Region have the same opportunities and facilities for diagnosis and treatment', and to achieve this it was necessary 'to get away from the idea of *ad hoc* local adjustment . . . and to concentrate on rationalisation on a broad regional basis', as had been done with infectious diseases hospitals. The SAMO went on to outline a method for doing this in the Hull and East Riding area, and asked the Board to make a decision on the principles involved in the method before any further attempts were made to reallocate beds to specialties.

The method used fell into three stages: first, the bed norms adopted by the medical advisory committees were used to calculate the beds required in each specialty in the Hull and East Riding area and the area as a whole; secondly, these figures were compared with existing provision and the percentage of need satisfied was computed; and, thirdly, a theoretical adjustment of bed allocation was made so that the same percentage of need was satisfied in each specialty and the area as a whole.

It may be helpful to illustrate this rather complicated methodology by using some examples from the report. On the medical advisory committees' standards, 82 gynaecological beds and 123 ENT beds were needed in Hull and East Riding. In fact, there were 111 gynaecological beds and 50 ENT beds, and so 135 per cent of need was satisfied in gynaecology and 41 per cent in ENT. The total number of beds in the area permitted 71 per cent of need to be satisfied in each specialty, and to equalise opportunities the allocation suggested was 58 in gynaecology (a reduction of 43), and 87 in ENT (an increase of 37). If applied to all specialties the same percentage of need – 71 per cent – would be satisfied. And, when reallocations had been made in each group, catchment areas could be altered so that the same need was satisfied between as well as within groups.

The SAMO stressed that acceptance of his proposals would not only equalise opportunities for treatment but would also help the Board in two other ways: first, the task of assessing the relative merits of applications from HMCs for capital expenditure would be simplified; and, secondly, in some cases the need for immediate in-patient and out-patient extensions at hospitals serving unnecessarily large areas would be obviated. The Board was asked 'to approve in principle the adoption of the theoretical allocation for each Group . . . as a yardstick in reviewing bed reallocations in management committee areas'.

After considerable discussion, the Board declined to give its approval. Instead, it 'received' the report, resolved that 'the proposals contained therein be not accepted', and decided to convene a meeting with the Hull and East Riding HMCs 'to assess, in the light of local conditions, the number of beds required for each specialty in each hospital'.

What reasons lay behind the rejection of the Plan?[6] First, it was argued that the application of uniform bed norms across the Region was misconceived because it failed to recognise that different areas had distinctive needs. For example, a district with a higher than average proportion of old people in the population would need more geriatric beds. This suggested that it was more important to pursue the goal of equitable provision than equal provision. Secondly, critics of the plan maintained that there was no sense in changing bed allocations if existing arrangements were satisfactory. These arrangements had to be studied carefully to see how well they were working before modifications were made, otherwise the result might be an unintended change for the worse. Thirdly, it was emphasised that reallocations had to be implemented incrementally rather than suddenly to allow time for adjustments in staffing and equipment to be made.

Finally, and most crucially, those who opposed the plan argued that it failed to take account of medico-political realities. In particular, the likely opposition of consultants, whose attitudes tend to be framed by concern with 'my work' and therefore 'my beds' and 'my unit', was felt to be a major barrier to the implementation of the proposals. To ask consultants to sacrifice beds to colleagues on the scale envisaged was perceived as unrealistic for it assumed an area consciousness which was just not present. Likewise, it was anticipated that there would be objections from local people, who grow accustomed to a particular pattern of provision and tend to resist changes propounded in the name of rationalisation. In short, the plan's critics maintained that the Board had to plan by consent, carrying with it medical staff and public opinion, and could not dictate from above what policy should be.

It was for these reasons that the plan was not accepted. Instead reallocations were made following consultation with staff and HMCs. The usual procedure was for the Board to submit proposals to HMCs, who, in association with their own medical advisory committees, would comment on the proposals and then meet the Board for discussions. While each set of proposals was drawn up in the light of local conditions, the principle of concentrating provision in specialties like ENT, obstetrics and gynaecology, ophthalmology, orthopaedic surgery and paediatrics in a single hospital in each district was applied throughout the Region. In some cases HMCs expressed their agreement with the Board's suggestions without holding a meeting; in other cases several meetings had to be convened before agreement could be reached. Wakefield fell into the latter category, and it was not until July 1956, more than four years after the Board had first considered bed reallocations in Wakefield, that proposals acceptable to the Board, HMCs and local medical staff were found. The main reason for the delay was opposition from consultants to any redistribution of beds, the SAMO reporting to the General Purposes Committee in 1953 that 'the detailed suggestions of the Medical Advisory Committee to the Wakefield "A" Group, with very minor exceptions, really amount to a continuation of the *status quo*'. This factor confirmed the views of those who had objected to the reallocation plan of October 1950.

Thus, decision-making on bed reallocation proceeded incrementally by means of 'partisan mutual adjustment'.[7] It was incremental in that each hospital group was dealt with individually and the changes which were agreed were small alterations to existing allocations. The principal partisans were the Board's medical officers and local medical staff, and the adjustments which were negotiated were a compromise between the more radical aspirations of the SAMO and his assistants and the more conservative inclinations of local consultants. This is in contrast to the original rational-comprehensive approach put forward by the SAMO, which was rational in the sense that it represented an 'ideal' solution to the uneven allocation of beds between specialties and areas, and comprehensive because it advocated a region-wide and specialty-wide approach. What happened in practice was that rather slower progress was made in reducing duplication and filling gaps in service provision. Nevertheless, the anticipated benefits of the pooling of beds in a district and regional system were beginning to accrue by the mid 1950s.

The years of make-do and mend

Turning now to the capital programme, the extent to which the Board could make good the shortage of beds noted in the Specialist Services Advisory Committee's survey depended on the amount of money made available by the Ministry of Health for new building. This amount in turn depended on the state of the national economy, and the decisions taken by central government on the distribution of public expenditure between different sectors. A complicating factor in the post-war period was the rationing of scarce building materials like steel and timber. In the event, priority was given to expenditure on schools, houses and defence, and hospitals had to take their place in the public expenditure queue. Up to 31 March 1953 only £46 million was expended on hospital fixed assets, an amount too small to permit anything more than a start to be made in meeting the need for capital development that had accumulated in the previous decade. As Titmuss and Abel-Smith later showed, as a proportion of gross fixed capital formation, hospital capital expenditure actually declined between 1949/1950 and 1953/1954, and in 1952/1953 was less than one-third of the level that obtained in 1938/1939.[8]

The paucity of capital funds posed considerable problems for regional boards. For example, in 1951 it was estimated that there were schemes to the value of £9.25 million of an 'urgent nature' needing to be carried out in the Leeds Region, yet up to 1953 actual capital expenditure was only £2 million. In this situation the Board necessarily concentrated on adaptations, conversions, reconditioning engineering services, and extending out-patient and diagnostic facilities. Thus, a former infectious diseases hospital at Oakwell, near Dewsbury, was converted for use by geriatric patients at a cost of £21 000; a pathology department was built at Kingston General Hospital, Hull, at a cost of £1600; and a new x-ray department was provided at Staincliffe General Hospital, Dewsbury, at a cost of £9300.

Well aware that the moneys allocated precluded boards from embarking on major schemes, in 1950 the Ministry of Health created a central reserve from which a limited number of projects costing over £100 000 could be financed. In the Leeds Region two such schemes were given the go-ahead: the former Emergency Medical Service hutted hospital at Fulford, York, was adapted for permanent use at a cost of £200 000; and a new 116-bed block was built at the Sutton Annexe of the Hull Royal Infirmary at a similar cost. However, cutbacks in public expenditure caused the central reserve to be abandoned in 1951, and this was one of the reasons why the Ministry refused the Board's application for funds to construct a new 300-bed sanatorium.

The priority the Board gave to this project is a reminder of the seriousness of tuberculosis in the first years of the NHS, a fact often overlooked twenty years later. The turning of the tide in the fight against the disease came in 1953, and from that year treatment with drugs like streptomycin and para-amino salicylic acid, the increasing use of domiciliary care, and more widespread BCG vaccination, rapidly and substantially reduced the need for further hospital accommodation. Indeed, in 1956 the Board set up a committee to advise on alternative uses of tuberculosis beds. In this case, then, the shortage of money for new building was a blessing in disguise, because, if the Board had started building a new sanatorium in the early 1950s, by the time it had come into operation it would have been surplus to requirements.

On the other hand, there were several urgently needed schemes, like the provision of additional accommodation at Huddersfield and Pontefract, which could not proceed due to lack of finance. As the Ministry of Health stated in its annual report for 1953:

> The main story of hospital capital development in the first five years of the National Health Service is of scarce resources carefully husbanded so as to bring the maximum results at the minimum cost, to make good as much damage and obsolescence as possible, and to provide modest extensions here and there where the need was greatest.[9]

Put another way, these were the years of 'make-do and mend', years when the patching up of existing hospitals took precedence over extensive new building.

Planning ahead

An indication that this period might be at an end came in 1954 when the Ministry asked boards for details of major projects which could be started in the following year if extra money became available. To its alarm, the Leeds Board discovered that none of its priority schemes was at a sufficiently advanced stage of planning to be submitted to the Ministry, and so it called for a review of 'the deficiencies and needs in the present hospital service in the Region and the priority with which such needs should be met'. The review, which was prepared by the Board's medical staff, was presented in two parts in June and October 1954, and it was the first major survey of hospital services since the Specialist Services Advisory Committee's survey of June 1949. As such, it recorded progress made in implementing that report, assessed existing deficiencies in different parts of the Region, and made recommendations for future developments.

The review began by noting the limitations that had been placed on the Board by the financial restriction of the previous six years. These restrictions notwithstanding, standards had been raised by 'modest works of improvement and modernisation', and the bed reallocation exercises had led to a more rational distribution of beds. It was therefore an opportune time 'to appraise the results and plan in detail for a further period, say of five years, whilst looking forward in broad outline for a much longer period'.

While both parts of the review were comprehensive in that they dealt with the whole range of hospital services – in-patient, out-patient and ancillary; acute and chronic; psychiatric and general – they concentrated on in-patient accommodation in the acute sector. In other words, a mixed scanning approach was again used. Since the Board had requested that deficiencies and needs should be identified, some means of comparing the position in different hospital districts had to be adopted. Bed norms were used for this purpose, but there was little evidence to indicate what these norms should be. The criterion used in the review was that the norms should be 'realistic and . . . likely to be attained in the foreseeable future', and a standard of 3.2 acute beds per thousand population was adopted.[10] Applied to the Region as a whole, this indicated a shortage of 1034 acute beds, with the deficiency being greatest in the Huddersfield, Pontefract and Keighley district hospital centres. Priority was therefore given to developments at those centres.

Shortly after the Board had completed its consideration of the review the Ministry of Health announced that a special fund was to be established to finance major works which boards could not carry out within their normal capital allocations. This initiative proved to be more soundly based than the short-lived central reserve introduced in 1950, and regular allocations were made from the fund until it was overtaken by the more ambitious programme contained in the Hospital Plan. Consequently, from 1955 onwards planning took on a new emphasis, becoming more and more concerned with the expanding building programme and less concerned with the rational-isation measures of the previous seven years. The main building projects undertaken in the Leeds Region were new hospitals at Huddersfield and Hull, and major improvements at Pontefract. The Keighley developments did not proceed because agreement could not be reached on whether the additional beds which were to be provided should be sited at Keighley or Skipton, towns separated by a distance of some ten miles.

By the end of the 1950s £1 million a year was being spent on hospital building in the Region, double the amount expended in the early years of the service. Capital expenditure had increased at the same rate nationally, reaching some £20 million a year in 1959/1960. Yet there were repeated demands for even greater expenditure, the most informed coming from Abel and Lewin, who, in a report prepared at the request of the BMA, argued for an expenditure of £750 million over ten years.[11] The Leeds Board received an indication that central government was taking these demands seriously in a report submitted by its officers in February 1960. The express intention of the report was 'to bring to the notice of the Board the need for urgent action in order that it will be able to cope with the anticipated large increase in the amount of moneys likely to be made available by the Minister of Health for expenditure upon capital projects'. A major expansion of the hospital building programme was thus signalled, and it seemed that after twelve years the NHS had reached the front of the public expenditure queue.

The Hospital Plan

The particular form that the expansion took was undoubtedly influenced by the coming together within the Ministry of Health in 1960 of Enoch Powell as Minister, Bruce Fraser as Permanent Secretary, and George Godber as Deputy Chief Medical Officer. These three men effectively transformed a vague idea about the need for an expanding building programme into a detailed development plan: *A Hospital Plan for England and Wales*, published in January 1962.[12] Fraser's role lay in negotiating with the Treasury for funds for a ten-year rolling programme – never an easy task. His success can be attributed partly to his personal skills and previous Treasury experience, but also it owed not a little to the idea of long-term planning of public expenditure, advocated at the time by the Plowden Committee.[13] Godber's role lay in stimulating boards into producing regional development plans. In 1960 Oxford and Wessex, at Godber's instigation, showed that regional plans were possible, and so in 1961 other regions were asked to follow suit. Powell's contribution was perhaps the most important, for he succeeded in welding these regional plans into a national Plan, played a major part in drafting the Plan, and ensured that it was published as a white paper.[14] Thus, although the Plan was very much the product of the work of hundreds of individuals throughout the country, its guiding principles and national character owed a great deal to the foresight of this triumvirate working at the centre of decision-making.

As already indicated, the Leeds Board began compiling its long term plan as early as February 1960, and over the next twelve months the officers prepared reports on developments needed in specific areas. It is interesting to note that it was around this time that the Board began using teams of medical and lay administrative staff and other officers to plan services, whereas prior to 1960 it had been the medical staff alone who had performed this function. Also, a number of 'commissions' of members were appointed to visit and report on hospitals in Hull, Bradford and York. In Leeds, which posed special problems because of the juxtaposition of teaching and regional hospitals, a joint working party of members had undertaken this task. A rather wider range of people was therefore involved in contributing to the Hospital Plan than previous planning exercises.

While the Board had available a good deal of information as a result of this work, the proposals put forward were more detailed and firmer in some areas than others. A comprehensive overview had been supplemented by specific plans for different parts of the Region. Thus, while the approach had again involved mixed scanning, the outcome was incremental, in that the plan which was submitted to the Ministry in May 1961 essentially involved building on past proposals and making successive small adjustments to the existing pattern of services. The plan's incrementalism was reinforced in the discussions which followed between Board officers and Ministry officials, the latter asking the Board to rethink a number of its more radical proposals, like the building of new small hospitals in places such as Goole, Selby and Otley.

The stated purpose of the Hospital Plan was:

> to give to the hospital service of England and Wales both the physical equipment and also the pattern and setting which will everywhere place the most modern treatment at the service of patients and enable the staffs who care for them to exercise their skill and devotion under the best conditions.[15]

The emphasis given to 'pattern and setting' as well as 'physical equipment' was deliberate, for the Plan not only contained details of major building works to be undertaken – 90 new and 134 substantially remodelled hospitals, together with a further 356 schemes costing over £100 000 each – but also provided a framework within which these works were to be carried out. At the centre of this framework was the district general hospital (DGH), a hospital normally of between 600 and 800 beds serving a population of

100 000–150 000, and providing all services except beds for mental subnormality and medium- and long-stay mental illness and facilities in regional specialties like plastic and thoracic surgery. It was a natural corollary of the development of a network of DGHs that many small hospitals would become redundant. The Plan did not refer much to hospital closures, but used the phrase 'as these schemes are completed, they will enable better provision to be made for the work now done at the following hospitals' to indicate the likely pattern of events.

Thus the main problem which was identified was the need to provide more modern accommodation rather than simply more accommodation. Overall, in fact, the number of beds provided was to be reduced, though this was accounted for mainly by the anticipated rundown of mental illness hospitals. To assist boards in planning future provision the Ministry laid down bed norms for acute, maternity, geriatric, mental illness and mental subnormality services. As the Plan acknowledged: 'There have hitherto been no generally accepted criteria for assessing the number of hospital beds of various kinds which are needed by a given population'.[16] It was therefore necessary to formulate criteria on the basis of the best available evidence in order that developments could proceed uniformly throughout the country. The norms proposed for acute (3.3/1000), maternity (0.58/1000) and mental subnormality (1.3/1000) beds caused little controversy. In contrast, the recommended norms for geriatric (1.4/1000) and mental illness (1.8/1000) beds were felt by many to be on the low side. The Ministry's answer to its critics was that in calculating these figures much greater provision of care outside hospital had been assumed. Indeed, the white paper emphasised that 'any plan for the development of the hospital service is complementary to the expected development of the services for prevention and for care in the community',[17] and a year after its publication a complementary white paper outlining local authorities' development proposals was published.

The main interest of these bed norms lies in the fact that they were the first attempt since 1948 to formulate national standards of provision. Moreover, they were all much lower than the 1948 norms and this can be explained partly by the unrealism of the earlier figures; partly by reductions in average lengths of stay and turnover intervals, which enabled more patients to be treated in fewer beds; and partly by the planned extension of community care. Similar norms had been used by boards in drawing up their plans, and the Ministry had insisted on these norms being followed: hence, another feature to note about the work which went into the Hospital Plan is that it was much more centrally guided and directed than previous planning exercises. By far the greatest part of the Plan was taken up with boards' proposals, and, although individual schemes were not costed, a total expenditure of £500 million in the ten years up to 1971 was envisaged, compared with an expenditure of £157 million in the first 13 years of the NHS. The Plan was therefore a major turning point, and established a pattern for the development of hospital services in the 1960s and beyond.

Implementing the Plan

In broad outline, the plan for the Leeds Region included the building of six new DGHs, and the extension and upgrading of several existing hospitals to DGH standard. The DGH concept was departed from only in Bridlington and Whitby, two of the more remote and less populous areas in the Region, where small new general hospitals were to be constructed. A new hospital was also proposed in the mental subnormality service, to be built at Wakefield. As far as mental illness services were concerned, there were to be extensions at a number of existing hospitals, major modernisation projects at others, and more widespread provision of general hospital units, but no new hospitals. Finally, new geriatric accommodation was to be provided in almost all parts of the Region. The total estimated cost of schemes expected to be started by the Board during the decade was £38.4 million.

These were the aspirations, but what happened in practice? In the first quinquennium of the Plan a number of the Board's major schemes were completed. These included the new Huddersfield Royal Infirmary, which started admitting patients in September 1966 and was the first entirely new hospital to be opened in the Region; the new Hull Royal Infirmary; major extensions at Pontefract General Infirmary; a variety of improvements at St James's Hospital, Leeds; a new ENT and eye unit at Bradford Royal Infirmary; the provision of additional mental illness beds and services at Lynfield Mount Hospital, Bradford, and Scalebor Park Hospital, Ilkley; and major redevelopments at St Luke's Hospital, Huddersfield, to provide acute, geriatric and psychiatric beds.

While these projects went ahead as planned, a number of the

Board's other schemes were either modified or dropped altogether. In Harrogate, for instance, where the initial plan was to extend Harrogate and District Hospital, it was discovered that the site was unsuitable for development, and so an alternative site was acquired in order that a completely new DGH could be built. In Dewsbury, the deliberately vague proposals contained in the Hospital Plan were made firmer by the Board's decision to develop Staincliffe General rather than Dewsbury General as the DGH for the area. Similarly, in Halifax the General Hospital rather than the Royal Infirmary was chosen as the hospital to be developed to provide a full range of services for the district. These changes and others were caused partly by new information revealed during more detailed planning and discussion; partly by alterations in the environment on which planning was imposed; and partly by political bargaining resulting in new adjustments and compromises.

With all these changes occurring at regional level, and with many of the schemes which did go ahead costing more than anticipated, it was becoming increasingly clear that a reappraisal of the Hospital Plan was needed, and in 1965 boards were called on to undertake such a reappraisal. The results were published in May 1966 as a white paper, *The Hospital Building Programme*.[18] This stated that the Hospital Plan's 'basic principles remain valid',[19] and it confirmed that there was to be no change in the bed norms set out in the Plan, nor in the concept of hospital services being based on DGHs. The white paper argued, however, that 'the expectations of the original Plan could not possibly have been fulfilled' because many of the schemes included in it were 'inadequately defined and imprecisely costed'.[20] Thus, although more money would be available – some £1000 million in the next decade – the Plan would have to proceed more slowly than had been envisaged. Above all, there was a need 'to bring greater realism to hospital planning'[21] and 'to get the best possible value for the resources provided'.[22] As the circular which initiated the reappraisal indicated, in some cases this would mean rebuilding the clinical core of existing hospitals, including x-ray departments, operating theatres, pathology laboratories and out-patient departments, leaving wards to be replaced at a later date, instead of the wholesale replacement of these hospitals.[23] Overall, then, there was much greater emphasis on precise costing, economy and value for money than in the original Plan.

This was reflected in the proposal to build an experimental district general hospital in the Leeds Region.[24] Arising out of its experience at St Luke's Hospital, Huddersfield, where an almost completely new 440-bed hospital for psychiatric, geriatric, maternity, medical and surgical patients was constructed at the low cost of £3100 a bed, the Board, in March 1963, commissioned the architects of the Huddersfield scheme, Poulsons, to determine whether a DGH could be designed at a comparably low cost. The architects and the Board's officers subsequently came up with a scheme to build 'a hypothetical peripheral general hospital' of 600 beds at an approximate cost of £4000 a bed. The Ministry responded enthusiastically to the Board's initiative and, with the assurance that finance for the project would be additional to the Region's expected capital allocation, invited the Board to make practical application of the principles contained in the scheme to an actual project in the Leeds Region.

The first requirement was to decide the location of the new hospital, and after considering the needs of several areas the Board came down in favour of the Keighley district. The district had two decisive advantages: it contained relatively weak medical interests, which was an important factor because it meant that these interests would not be clamouring for their own special needs to be catered for in the new hospital; and, secondly, because of the horizontal layout of the hospital a large flat site was needed, and it was anticipated that one could be found in the district. This indeed proved possible, and a site acceptable to the HMC and local authorities was acquired at Eastburn, midway between Keighley and Skipton. Detailed planning then began, with most of the work being done by the Board's planning team and a special team set up by the Ministry, both teams comprising mainly medical, nursing, architectural, engineering and administrative officers. The architects and group secretary were intimately involved at all stages, and the Board's planning team held several meetings with the HMC and local medical staff. Instead of exchanging correspondence, the teams from the Board and Ministry met regularly and this greatly expedited the planning process. The result was that the final cost limit was submitted to the Ministry in December 1964, only 13 months after approval in principle had been given to the scheme; work on site commenced in September 1966; and the hospital was opened to patients in May 1970, just over seven years after it had been conceived. This was a remarkably short time, and was due in no small part to the fact that the Eastburn project was used by the Ministry as the testing ground for new planning procedures later applied more generally as the National Health Service Capital Projects Code (CAPRICODE).

Apart from the speed with which the scheme was carried out, the project was also noteworthy for its cost. Although this rose sharply from the original estimate, the eventual cost of around £9000 a bed compared favourably with other hospitals built at the same time. One of the main reasons for this was the horizontal layout. Whereas the new Huddersfield and Hull hospitals were built upwards, Eastburn was based on a two-storey design in which one of the principal aims was the reduction of 'on-costs', or costs rising from the way a site is used. Thus, the hospital formed the shape of a cross, each of the four arms of the cross containing departments of similar function: medical, surgical, geriatric and psychiatric wards were in the western arm; maternity, paediatric and private wards in the southern arm; ancillary departments in the eastern arm; and service and supply departments in the northern arm. Departments using steam were thereby grouped together, and were located next to the source of supply. Standardisation was used wherever possible, and the wards, for instance, each accommodated thirty beds divided into two wings comprising three 4-bed bays and three single wards. The extensive application of industrialised building techniques and materials was another feature of the project. These factors combined to reduce overall costs and, while the completed hospital may have lacked aesthetic merit, it was very definitely value for money.

Viewed in the national context, Eastburn was of interest because it epitomised the change in emphasis expressed in the 1966 Hospital Building Programme. As we have seen, the Programme made clear that the Hospital Plan had been over-optimistic. In order to secure the replacement of old and unsatisfactory hospitals as rapidly as possible, building costs had to be reduced to a minimum. One reason why costs were so high was that each new hospital was planned on a tailor-made basis, with the different professional groups involved in hospital work each wanting a say in how the cloth was cut. Also the involvement of these groups increased the design time, which further pushed up costs. The development of Building Notes, published by the Ministry from 1961 onwards, was an attempt to introduce an element of standardisation, but Eastburn went much further, and it was the forerunner of the 'Best Buy' projects at Bury St Edmunds and Frimley.[25] Its significance was therefore national as well as regional and local, and the initiative the Board took in proposing the scheme and the support the Ministry gave to that initiative showed that innovation and experimentation were possible in hospital planning.

Big is beautiful?

The search for economy and efficiency which lay behind the Eastburn scheme also figured prominently in the Bonham-Carter report, 'The Functions of the District General Hospital',[26] published in 1969. This report took the DGH concept to its ultimate conclusion in suggesting that on grounds of efficiency, and in order to reap the full benefits of economies of scale, a DGH should be based on teams of not less than two consultants in each specialty. Most DGHs should therefore be planned to serve populations of between 200 000 and 300 000 instead of 100 000–150 000 as previously. Further, the report recommended that provision for mental illness, mental handicap and geriatrics should be integrated into DGHs, and that 'small hospitals should be retained only as "peripheral hospital *units*" '[27] (emphasis added) with a strictly limited role. A review of the hospital building programme was called for, to bring the programme into line with these recommendations.

The report was received less than enthusiastically. Immediate evidence of this was contained in the prefatory note by the Secretary of State for Social Services and the Secretary of State for Wales, who stated that the report's recommendations 'should help to stimulate discussion', but added:

> Before conclusions can be reached on its findings and recommendations they will have to be further considered in the light of the likely future pattern of community health and social services. In particular a lot more thought must be given to the best way of providing for people who need long-term care, and also to the functions of smaller hospitals supplementary to the district general hospitals.[28]

The Central Health Services Council also drew attention to the significance of smaller hospitals in its foreword to the report, noting 'the potentially important complementary role of the "peripheral hospital units" '.[29] Other observers pointed out the inconvenience to patients of further concentrating hospital services, and argued that the Bonham-Carter committee had failed to take proper account of the social costs of its recommendations. For these reasons the concept of the very large DGH quickly came under attack.

Hospital planners were constantly being reminded of the social costs of their decisions in the late 1960s. In particular, the closure of small hospitals, which invariably accompanied the completion of new developments, was often strongly resisted by the communities in which these hospitals were situated. The Leeds Board had frequent first hand experience of such resistance, most notably in the opposition it encountered when the closure of the Adela Shaw Hospital at Kirkbymoorside was proposed. Of the 96 beds at this orthopaedic hospital, only 60 were occupied, and of this number only 10 were occupied by people from the immediately surrounding area. As a result of improvements to hospitals in Scarborough the Board proposed the closure of the hospital, and when this became known local residents organised to oppose the proposal: an action committee was formed; the support of the MP for the area was enlisted; and the local authorities concerned expressed their opposition to the closure. Following a packed public meeting in Kirkbymoorside in July 1968 attended by senior Board officers and members, the Board reaffirmed its policy, and the Secretary of State subsequently agreed to the hospital being closed.

Kirkbymoorside was not an isolated case, and a year later resistance to closure proposals had reached such a level that the Board's chairman took the unusual step of making a statement at the bi-monthly meeting of the Board clarifying the policy of concentrating services in DGHs. DHSS was equally concerned at the extent of public feeling, and in 1969 introduced a new procedure for hospital closures designed to involve the public at a much earlier stage in the decision making process. As one of the Department's senior officials put it, the purpose of the procedure was

> to get a very much better system of public relations and to make sure consultations are carried out properly. I think there have been cases in the past where consultations have perhaps not been all that they might have been, or they have been carried out too late.[30]

At around the same time boards were given general authority to appoint information officers, a measure also intended to improve public relations. These developments, which were very much in line with attempts to increase public participation in fields like local authority planning,[31] began the process of opening up hospital planning to a wider public.

Viewed against this background it was not surprising that the Bonham-Carter report was received with reservations. However, the response from DHSS to the report was ambiguous, and in the absence of anything but general murmurings that the report's proposals were not entirely acceptable, planners in the Leeds Region continued much as before: work started on new DGHs at Harrogate and York in 1971; existing hospitals in Dewsbury, Halifax, Pontefract and Scarborough were steadily upgraded to DGH standard; and major improvements were carried out at St James's Hospital, Leeds, which in 1970 was designated a university hospital in recognition of its increasing role in medical education.

The only area affected in a significant way by the Bonham-Carter report was Bradford, where the Board decided to develop one large DGH around the existing Royal Infirmary, instead of building a new DGH to operate in conjunction with the Infirmary, as was proposed in the Hospital Plan. However, it was not until 1971, after lengthy consultations with officials of DHSS and the Secretary of State, that the Bradford Corporation agreed to this change of policy, by which time the Bradford developments had been deferred in the building programme and their place taken by the new DGH at York.

At the opposite end of the scale plans continued to be developed for two small new hospitals at Bridlington and Whitby. Because of their isolated and scattered populations these areas did not fit easily into the district general hospital network, and so local hospital provision had to be made. Part of the reaction against the 'big is beautiful' philosophy epitomised by the Bonham-Carter report was a renewal of interest in the functions of small hospitals, and attention centred on the 'community hospital' concept pioneered in the Oxford Region.[32] As it emerged in the early 1970s, this concept involved the provision of a unit staffed primarily by GPs and usually containing out-patient clinics, a geriatric day hospital, a small number of geriatric, general and maternity beds, and elementary diagnostic facilities. This in essence was the type of hospital the Leeds Board had been planning for Whitby since publication of the Hospital Plan, except that it also contained a health centre and as such was an interesting example of integrated health services planning. A somewhat larger hospital was planned for Bridlington.

Although DHSS did not officially endorse the provision of

community hospitals until August 1974, for some time before then the Department had made clear to boards its interest in the concept. And the reasons for this were as much social and political as medical. Community hospitals were seen to be 'more convenient for patients, visitors and staff'; they were valued by local people, as was evidenced by the resistance encountered when the closure of small hospitals was proposed; and they were needed for patients who did not require the specialised facilities of district general hospitals, yet who could not be cared for in their own homes.[33] Thus, after a period of ambiguity, the future of small, local hospitals became more certain.

The expanding building programme benefited psychiatric and geriatric services as well as general hospital services. Indeed, one of the largest schemes carried out by the Board was the building of a new 480-bed hospital for the mentally handicapped at Wakefield, opened to patients in 1972. New accommodation was also provided in the mental illness service, including the provision of units in the general hospitals at Eastburn and Halifax, and a small unit at St. Mary's Hospital, Scarborough, which brought local psychiatric facilities to the area for the first time. But it was in the geriatric service that the greatest progress was made, with new accommodation being provided in almost all parts of the Region. Among the many schemes which went ahead were a new 192-bed hospital at Bierley Hall, Bradford, a 256-bed geriatric unit in the new Northowram Hall Hospital, Halifax, a new 192-bed hospital at Newton Green, Leeds, and a 120-bed unit at Castleford, Normanton and District Hospital. At the same time there was a marked increase in geriatric day hospital provision. Increasingly old unsatisfactory accommodation was replaced by purpose-built hospitals as plans laid in the early 1960s reached fruition ten years later; and, as we indicate in Chapter 5, 13 per cent of the Board's capital budget was spent on geriatric services between 1969 and 1974.

In short, in the 12 years after publication of the Hospital Plan there were major improvements in the standard of accommodation in all sectors of the hospital service. And while, as we have shown, there were changes and delays in some of the proposals contained in the Plan, many of the schemes put forward in 1962 were carried through. If a balance sheet were drawn up it would show that by 1974 of the major DGH developments all but two – those at Bradford and Leeds – were either completed or were well under way; that planning for the new small hospitals at Bridlington and Whitby was at an advanced stage and in the case of Whitby was brought to fruition after 1974; and that the vast majority of the developments planned in long-stay services, modest as these were in some cases, were implemented.

However, hospital capital expenditure reached a peak in 1973/1974, the last year of the Board's existence, and thereafter declined as a result of public expenditure cuts caused by national economic problems. The period of retrenchment which followed, characterised by some as a return to the era of 'make-do and mend' of the 1950s, in retrospect made the years 1962–74 seem like the golden age of hospital building. The inescapable consequence was that after 1974 'many much needed new hospitals and other developments will not be able to proceed . . . and the size of other projects will have to be reduced and their timetables extended.'[34] The way in which planners responded to this challenge lies outside the period of the present study. However, as the past often holds pointers to the future, it may be useful to summarise and analyse the experience of planning hospital and specialist services in the Leeds Region between 1948 and 1974.

Conclusion

In trying to make sense of the Board's experience as a planning agency, it may be helpful to return to the questions set out at the beginning of this chapter. The first question was: *Who was involved?* The evidence presented here demonstrates that the main participants in planning were the Board's officers, and that up to 1960 it was the medical officers, in conjunction with senior medical staff in the Region's hospitals, who dominated planning. After that date the circle of participants widened to include Board members, who had had a limited involvement before then, and other officers. Direct participation by the public was limited to protests over hospital closures, while indirectly the public's views were heard via Board and HMC members, and through any influence local authorities were able to bring to bear. The involvement of the Ministry of Health, and later DHSS, varied. Up to the Hospital Plan, the Ministry adopted a *laissez-faire* approach with regard to hospital planning, apparently content to let boards plan within their centrally allocated capital budgets, and not intervening to ensure conformity with national guidelines or to influence regional priorities. The only limited exception was in relation to psychiatric services, where a small central fund known as the 'mental million' was created in the mid 1950s.[35] Otherwise, boards exercised their planning responsibilities with a fair measure of autonomy, as indicated by the absence of any generally accepted bed norms. This changed in 1960, when work started on preparing the Hospital Plan. Recommended bed norms were circulated to boards, and the expanding building programme became much more centrally guided. Yet the extent of central involvement should not be overemphasised. Although it was demonstrably greater than in the 1950s, boards still had considerable freedom within the broad limits imposed by national budgets and guidelines. As we discuss in Chapter 8, the development and implementation of the Hospital Plan is best seen as a period when the Ministry and boards moved forward together.

The second question was: *What approach to planning was used?* What we hope to have shown is that the dominant approach was mixed scanning, or an approach which lay somewhere between rational-comprehensiveness and incrementalism. The only attempt to plan on a rational-comprehensive basis was the SAMO's bed reallocation exercise of 1950, but this foundered on the rock of medical objections. Otherwise, the method used involved a broad scan of the whole range of hospital and specialist services followed by more detailed study of particular areas or problems. Yet, if the approach approximated to comprehensiveness, the outcome was almost invariably incremental. The strength of existing interests, particularly medical interests, made small adjustments the limit of what was possible. Exceptions served only to prove the rule, as the complete reorganisation of infectious diseases hospitals, where medical interests were weak, showed.

Thirdly: *How was the problem defined?* The initial review of services carried out in 1948 and 1949 defined the main problems facing the Board as being the shortage and maldistribution of beds, and the poor quality of much of the hospital stock. Other problems identified were the wasteful dispersal of beds between hospitals, inadequate and insufficient out-patient and ancillary facilities, and lack of co-ordination of infectious diseases hospitals. Many of these problems remained on the agenda throughout the period, although some, like the bed shortage, were seen to be a chimera, while others, like the coordination of infectious diseases hospitals, were satisfactorily tackled. Above all, the need to concentrate beds in a smaller number of new hospitals continued to be a prominent policy goal.

This leads into the fourth question: *What was the policy response*? We have shown that the main response of planners was to work up a building programme, and only at the beginning and the end of the period was this not true. In the early years of the NHS the shortage of funds for building meant that attention was focussed on improvements which involved little or no expenditure, like the extension of out-patient services or the realignment of existing facilities. Again, towards the end of the period, in April 1968 and October 1971, the Board published a 'Review of Policy and Objectives' which took services as its starting point and, after outlining expected trends in staffing, ancillary, and other relevant services, detailed developments which were to occur in each area of the Region over a three-year period. Although the emphasis was still on new building, the fact that the Reviews even considered other variables was a significant departure from past practice.

Nevertheless, it was capital planning rather than service planning which dominated the Board's activities and it is not difficult to find the reason why. In carrying out their reviews and surveys, the Board's planners usually started by asking which areas had a shortage of beds or a large proportion of beds in unsuitable accommodation, and then proceeded to identify building priorities. Only rarely were units other than the bed used to compare hospital provision in different areas, and considerable effort was put into devising bed norms for the Region and the country as a whole. If other units had been used – for example, waiting times for treatment, length of stay and turnover intervals – then planning might have developed in different directions.

The 1966 Hospital Building Programme explicitly acknowledged that there were alternatives to the provision of additional beds and that 'the significance of the bed as the unit for measuring the hospital provision required can be exaggerated'.[36] It argued that improvements to ancillary facilities and the more widespread use of day-patient and out-patient treatment could improve the quality of hospital services just as much as the provision of extra accommodation. How far this move was prompted by a pragmatic recognition that the resources available for capital building would never be sufficient to meet all demands, and how far it was based on a conviction that new patterns of provision were likely to be more effective, is not known, but the move was strengthened by the emergence of the idea of service planning in the late 1960s.

According to Barnard, 'as a general principle, the intentions of service planning are that the emphasis should be on service and not on the particular vehicles or means that are used to provide the service'[37]: hence, decision-makers ask what pattern of services they wish to provide, and then decide 'the means that are needed in order for such a pattern of services to exist – buildings, equipment, types of manpower and the rest. Decisions on capital development would then emerge as outputs of the planning process – not the determining factor.'[38] As we have noted, while these ideas had an influence on the Leeds Board's planning activities towards the end of its life, for the most part planning was synonymous with the capital building programme.

Moving on from this, the next question is: *How was the Board's policy implemented*? In recent years writers interested in policy analysis have turned their attention to issues of implementation, their concern often being shaped by a perceived 'failure' by government to achieve its stated goals.[39] However, it is important to balance the 'top-down' model of the policy process implied by the word implementation, with an examination of the other side of the coin, innovation. How far, in other words, do planning systems encourage innovation at the local level? The one major example of innovation in the Leeds Region was the new hospital at Eastburn, which has been discussed in some detail. Examples from elsewhere, like the development of community hospitals in the Oxford Region, show that the capacity to innovate was not unique to Leeds. Both instances indicate that there was sufficient autonomy at board level for this kind of initiative to emerge, and that the central department gave sufficient encouragement for them to get off the ground.

As far as implementation is concerned, our data show that the Board achieved a high 'success' rate in implementing its policies. And this is not surprising. If, as we have argued, the main emphasis were on new building in the context of an expanding capital programme, then it might be anticipated that there would be a high degree of congruence on objectives and goals. After all, nobody objects to new hospitals. People do sometimes object to the siting of new hospitals, however, and it was this which caused delay in the new building planned for Keighley and Bradford. In both cases local authority opposition caused the Board's plans to be deferred, though not reversed. Implementation problems arose most clearly, though, when it came to reallocating existing services and resources and closing hospitals. The most striking example was the bed reallocation exercise conducted throughout the 1950s, where the strength of entrenched medical interests was a source of often substantial opposition and delay to the Board's proposals. A more general point follows: that in the NHS the existence of powerful professional interests at the operational level is likely to be the main obstacle to the implementation of agreed policies.

This begins to suggest an answer to the penultimate question: *Whose will prevailed*? Here it may be helpful to refer to the work of Robert Alford, who in a study of health planning in New York identifies what he calls three sets of 'structural interests': these are the professional monopolisers, who are the dominant interests; the corporate rationalisers, who are the challenging interests; and the community population, who are the repressed interests.[40] This typology fits the data presented here very well: we have already drawn attention to the lack of public involvement in hospital planning in the Leeds Region, and to the way in which attempts to rationalise services were sometimes frustrated by professional interests. Indeed, the history of hospital planning between 1948 and 1974 can be seen as the history of corporate rationalisers, represented by regional board planners, trying to challenge the established interests of the medical profession, with the community hardly in earshot. Of course, this is an oversimplified picture of the world and it would be wrong to see these interests as entirely homogeneous and always opposed to one another. For example, the Bonham-Carter report can be seen as an alliance between the interests of the professional monopolisers and corporate rationalisers against community interests, but the outcome demonstrates the ability of policy-makers within DHSS to defend successfully community interests. Again, divisions among professional monopolisers often provide a more important dynamic in the policy-making process than divisions between interests. Nevertheless, the picture which has been painted here has a high level of descriptive validity. What our data show is that, while the corporate rationalisers made some impact into medical hegemony, their progress was slow and incremental. The absence of overt conflict helped to sustain the position of the medical profession for, as Alford reminds us, dominant interests are served by existing social, economic and political institutions. In the words of another writer, there is in all political systems a 'mobilisation of bias'[41] in favour of some interests, which means that unless they are challenged these interests continue to dominate. This implies that, simply by virtue of their known or anticipated power, dominant interests will rule some issues off the agenda and control others by non-decision-making. And this, we have argued, is why the only radical challenge to the medical profession's interests made by corporate rationalisers in the Leeds Board – the major bed reallocation plan put forward in 1950 – was rejected.

We are now on the way to answering the final question: *Who benefited*? The medical profession were clear beneficiaries, as measured by improved facilities, additional equipment, more modern buildings, and so on, although it should be noted that a theme of later chapters is that some groups within the profession were more successful than others in the struggle for scarce resources. The community also benefited from these improvements, apart from the

TABLE 3.1   *Proportion of capital expenditure allocated to each HMC,*
1948–74

Leeds (St James's) University	12.97
Hull 'A'	11.90
Huddersfield	10.53
York 'A'	7.71
Airedale	7.53
Bradford	7.16
Wakefield	6.49
Halifax	5.74
Pontefract, Castleford and Goole	5.44
Harrogate and Ripon	4.82
Leeds 'B'	4.11
East Riding	2.72
Dewsbury, Batley and Mirfield	2.62
Scarborough, Bridlington, Malton and Whitby	2.62
Hull 'B'	2.55
York 'B'	2.17
Wharfedale	2.00
High Royds	0.92
Total	**100.00**

SOURCE   Leeds RHB, *Expenditure on Capital Works* (Harrogate, 1974). Excludes expenditure on Board HQ, regional services and hospitals closed, which together comprised nearly 7 per cent of this total.

disbenefits to patients and their families which arose when small, local hospitals were closed. There are two other measures of who benefited, both based on an analysis of capital expenditure. The first concerns the distribution of expenditure between different types of hospital. What this demonstrates is that by far the highest proportion – 64 per cent – was spent on general hospitals; 6.5 per cent on geriatric hospitals; 8 per cent on mental illness hospitals; 6.5 per cent on mental handicap hospitals; and the remainder – 15 per cent – on other hospitals and services.[42] The second measure concerns the distribution of expenditure between different areas, and the relevant data are presented in Table 3.1. They show, not surprisingly, that the areas to benefit most were Leeds, Hull and Huddersfield, where there was a major investment in general hospital services. It will be recalled that the initial review of services carried out by the Board had identified Hull and Huddersfield as being the most deprived in the Region, and so there was a certain logic in this expenditure pattern. Again not surprisingly, the areas to benefit least were those which contained a preponderance of long-stay hospitals. Expenditure distribution is, however, only one way of measuring the area allocation of resources, and in the next chapter we examine how the distribution of senior medical staff changed throughout the period.

4

Medical Staffing

The wartime Hospital Surveys identified the shortage and maldistribution of consultants and specialists as one of the main shortcomings of the hospital service before the advent of the NHS. In this chapter we examine how this problem was tackled, focusing on the distribution of consultants between regions and within the Leeds Region, changes in the medical staffing structure, and the various attempts to plan medical manpower. This by no means exhausts the list of possible topics which might be covered, but it does reflect the items which occupied the time of the Leeds Board. Consideration of these issues also illustrates more general questions about planning and policy making in the NHS.

By way of introduction, it is worth going back to the report of the Spens Committee, which reported in 1948 on the pay of hospital doctors.[1] The Committee recommended that there should be five grades of medical staff in hospitals, organised in the form of a competitive training ladder. The aspiring consultant would have to progress from a house officer post through the junior registrar (later re-named senior house officer), registrar and senior registrar grades before achieving his goal. Training for a consultant post was expected to take approximately seven years, although at any time a trainee might 'fall off the training ladder' and into general practice. The structure recommended by the Spens Committee was accepted by the medical profession, with the addition of the senior hospital medical officer (SHMO) and junior hospital medical officer (JHMO) grades. Both grades were of unlimited tenure and outside the training ladder, and were intended as a temporary measure to meet the needs of doctors already working in the hospital service who lacked the qualifications to be included in the main staffing structure. In all, then, there were seven hospital doctor grades, as well as the part-time clinical assistant grade designed for GPs wishing to participate in hospital work.

For this structure to work effectively, there needed to be considerably more consultants than junior doctors in training. If the seven-year training period were adhered to, then consultants would remain in post for thirty years or more, and it has been estimated that 'for all career intentions to be fulfilled there must be between three and five times as many consultant posts as there are junior posts'.[2] The ratio would be reduced if, as was highly likely, some junior doctors left for general practice, emigrated, or for other reasons did not complete their training. Even so, the message was clear: a balanced staffing structure was a top-heavy staffing structure.

In the early years of the NHS there were grounds for believing that this might be achieved. In the Leeds Region many new consultant posts were created after September 1949. Up to that date only a handful of appointments were made because it was not clear how many existing consultant staff there were in the Region. The task of deciding in which grades in the new staffing structure doctors should be employed was given to a 'status committee' which had as its nucleus two general physicians, two general surgeons, and one obstetrician and gynaecologist. The committee was subsequently enlarged by the addition of representatives of the Royal Colleges and external assessors to hear appeals against its decisions. Only when the committee's work was complete did the Leeds Board advertise new posts, and the general aim of Board policy was to establish teams of consultants in general surgery, general medicine, obstetrics and gynaecology, paediatrics, pathology, ENT, opthalmology, radiology, anaesthetics, short-stay orthopaedic surgery and geriatrics at each of the district hospital centres in the Region. Although precise figures are not available, we have estimated that between 1948 and 1952 there was a 50 per cent increase in the number of consultant sessions carried out in the Region, and this increase permitted the more obvious gaps in service provision to be filled.[3]

At the same time there was a large expansion of the junior grades, resulting from the creation by HMCs of new house officer and registrar posts. While these junior doctors were needed to staff the hospital service, the numbers employed threatened the Spens training ladder concept. That is, there were more doctors on the middle rungs of the ladder than could be absorbed into the consultant grade in the time expected, despite the expansion of the consultant grade. This was a cause of concern to both the Leeds Board and the Ministry of Health.

A report to the Board in January 1950 recommended that registrar and senior registrar establishments should be limited to the number of consultant vacancies likely to be available, and this was accepted. In September of the same year the Ministry transferred the power to appoint registrars from HMCs to RHBs, who were in a better position to assess manpower needs. Two months later a circular was issued which stated that on the assumption that there were likely to be 150 consultant vacancies annually in England and Wales in the coming years, the number of senior registrar posts should be limited to 600 and registrar posts to 1100. The recommended total of 1700 was 1100 less than the number of registrars in post in 1950.[4]

These proposals caused grave disquiet in the medical profession, which raised the spectre of hundreds of redundant registrars. Negotiations were hurriedly arranged, and in September 1951 the Ministry sent revised proposals to regional boards: no formal limit was to be placed on the number of registrar posts, which was to be fixed by each board according to local needs and conditions; the trainee concept was modified by making the registrar grade a staffing grade instead of a training grade; the senior registrar establishment was increased from 600 to 960; and the training period of senior registrars was extended from three years to four.[5]

Here, then, was a classic example of a rational approach to manpower planning being overturned by political objections. Rationally, there was no doubt that the number of junior doctors had to be reduced, if the staffing structure were not to be imbalanced; politically, the medical profession made it clear that redundancies among junior doctors were unacceptable. The outcome represented a clear victory for the professional monopolisers over the corporate rationalisers. One of the consequences was that a bottleneck appeared in the training ladder, with the result that many senior registrars remained in post five years or more before being appointed consultants. As Godber later acknowledged: 'This in retrospect was one of the least wise actions or pieces of inaction in the early 1950s. The control of senior registrars introduced in 1952 was not enough . . .'[6]

One of the interesting aspects of this case is that the problem was defined as too many junior doctors, rather than too few consultants.

Clearly, one way around the bottleneck would have been to have expanded the consultant grade. For reasons of cost this was not done, and in fact in December 1952 central control of consultant establishments was introduced, and thereafter there was a considerable reduction in the rate of increase of consultant staff.[7] Inevitably this accentuated the plight of junior doctors, and it illustrated that the corporate rationalisers did have some control over manpower policy. These moves, though, can also be seen to be in the interests of senior members of the medical profession, whose bargaining power in wage negotiations might have been reduced if their numbers had been increased more rapidly. The interests of junior and senior hospital doctors did not always coincide, and this is a point we discuss further below.

In making new consultant appointments after 1949, the Leeds Board used as a general guide the staffing standards worked out by its medical advisory committees. These standards detailed the number and type of consultant sessions required in each hospital group, and as such they were potentially an important means of overcoming the maldistribution of staff. In 1955 revised standards were put forward for the consideration of the Board by the SAMO. The SAMO's report was interesting because in many ways it paralleled his 1950 report on bed reallocation, discussed in Chapter 3, in that it sought a comprehensive and rational approach to planning. The report began by noting the difficulty of laying down rigid staffing standards 'in view of the number of variables which affect the position in each hospital or hospital group'. It continued, 'nevertheless in each specialty a certain broad pattern has emerged', and went on to show how revised standards in 'two fairly typical specialties' – orthopaedic surgery and ENT – could be calculated on the basis of population served and available beds, the same criteria as were used in 1949. These standards were intended to 'serve solely as a general guide to the Staff and Establishments Committee in considering applications for additional sessions or for new appointments, and in assessing relative needs in the Region', and when applied to orthopaedic surgery and ENT they showed no need for major changes. The report concluded by asking the Board to approve in principle the technique employed, adding that if this were done standards in other specialties would be reviewed.

The Board referred the report to its main medical advisory committee, the Specialist Services Advisory Committee, which drew particular attention to the effect of local facilities on the output of a consultant. As the report had recognised, this made the precise definition of standards extremely difficult. Accordingly, because of the numerous variables affecting individual appointments, the Committee felt that it was not possible to improve on the standards agreed in 1949, and the Board accepted this advice. Thereafter each request for a new consultant appointment was investigated and argued in the light of the local situation, and the standards declined in importance. As the Board explained in evidence to the Royal Commission on Doctors' and Dentists' Remuneration, its view was that 'extra posts should be agreed as a result of the study of the work of the hospitals and clinics in the area and not by the hard and fast application of theoretical standards'. In other words, just as in the case of the bed reallocation proposals, an incremental rather than a rational comprehensive approach was used, with the views of the professional monopolisers again winning out over those of the corporate rationalisers.

The distribution of consultants

Requests for extra consultant posts came from a variety of sources, including HMCs, group and regional medical advisory committees, and the Board's own medical officers. When submitted to the Ministry these requests had to be supported by a detailed statement of need which referred to such variables as length of waiting list, bed occupancy and turnover, available facilities, and additional expenditure entailed. An Advisory Committee on Consultant Establishments was set up by the Ministry to consider boards' applications, but the Committee's role was essentially reactive. As Stevens has noted, the Committee 'was not primarily intended to redistribute senior hospital medical staff. Its chief function was to ration the available supply of consultants in the face of increasing demands from employing boards'.[8] There were, in any case, no nationally agreed staffing standards which the Committee could use to assess the priority of boards' demands or to attempt to equalise the distribution of consultants. Consequently, the inequalities which existed between regions were perpetuated and in some cases increased, and we discuss this further below.

But what happened within regions? This is an issue on which very little information has hitherto been presented. Eckstein admits that the situation is 'obscure' and without supporting evidence goes on to claim that 'at least developments have been in the right direction';[9] in a similar vein Ryan says that in 1958 the Welsh Hospital Board 'could claim to have achieved an appropriate geographical distribution' of consultants, but again does not present any supporting figures;[10] and Stevens comments that an analysis of the distribution of specialists within regions does not 'lend[s] itself easily to statistical measurement', because 'consultant statistics are published only on a regional basis'.[11]

However, by gathering information from a number of published and unpublished sources it has been possible to make an assessment of changes in the distribution of consultants within the Leeds Region between 1948 and 1960, and 1960 and 1972.[12] The findings are illustrated in Figures 4.1 and 4.2, which show the variation from the regional average of areas within the Region. The variation has been expressed in terms of consultant sessions per 100 000 population, which is the usual way of expressing the distribution of medical staff. What the figures demonstrate is a striking reduction in the inequalities which existed in 1948. In that year the variation in consultant sessions between areas was from 76 per cent below the regional average to 53 per cent above, while in 1960 the variation was from 37 per cent below the regional average to 31 per cent above. After 1960 there was some deterioration in the distribution, and in 1972 the variation between areas ranged from 40 per cent below the regional average to 43 per cent above. Some of the variations which remained can be explained by complementarity between areas. The well-endowed Wakefield area, for example, also served the poorly-endowed Pontefract area. This highlights one of the main limitations of the data: the populations on which the figures are based are those adopted by the Board for planning purposes and, although these populations take some account of cross-boundary patient flows, it is doubtful if they take full account of these flows. The effect of regional specialties and teaching hospital provision on consultant staffing also have to be borne in mind.[13] It is clear, for instance, that the high staffing ratio in Leeds owed much to the presence within the area of the teaching hospital and associated regional specialty centres. Despite the limitations of the data, the overriding impression is of a considerable evening-up in the distribution of consultants within the Region. This supports Stevens' assessment that 'the build-up of "peripheral" consultant services, or those away from the major

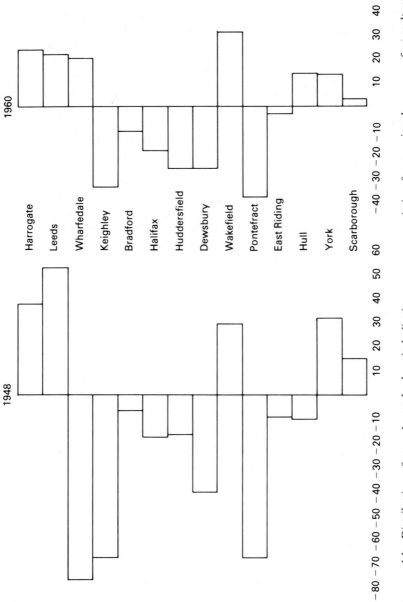

FIGURE 4.1 Distribution of consultants by hospital district – percentage variation from regional average of consultant sessions per 100 000 population

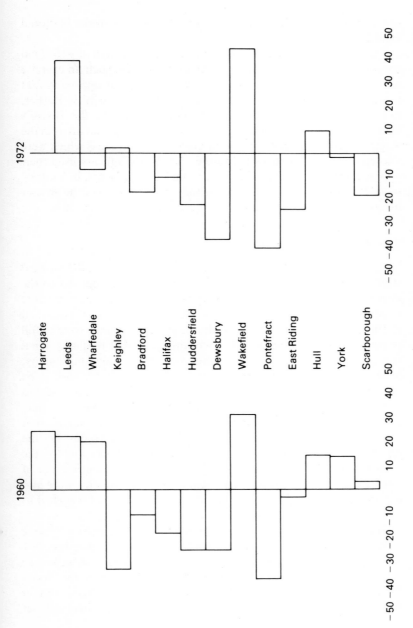

FIGURE 4.2 Distribution of consultants by hospital district – percentage variation from regional average of consultant sessions per 100 000 population

towns in the region, is perhaps the greatest success in the National Health Service'.[14]

The Leeds Board achieved this 'success' not through any rational comprehensive planning exercise. As we have seen, such an exercise was rejected in favour of an incremental, case by case, approach. Yet this approach did not simply involve 'muddling through'.[15] Rather, it took the form of guided incrementalism, in that the Board's medical officers used their detailed knowledge of different areas in the Region to push for new consultant posts in certain areas which were known to be most deficient. In other words, the officers used their appreciation of medical manpower to make judgements, in Vickers' sense,[16] about priorities. It was this that enabled some of the grosser inequalities in the distribution of consultants to be overcome.

The Platt working party

By the end of the 1950s the continuing problems with the medical staffing structure and the Spens training ladder concept led to the appointment of the Platt working party, asked to advise on how the structure might be improved. The working party's report, published in 1961, recommended that consultants should continue to take full responsibility for patients.[17] The working party felt that additional consultants were needed, but did not attempt to assess how many, instead recommending that special review committees should be established in each region to survey staffing needs and submit proposals for extra posts. The retention of the senior registrar grade, primarily as a training grade, was advocated, as was the retention of the registrar, senior house officer and house officer grades. On the other hand, the working party favoured the phasing out of the SHMO and JHMO grades. In the place of the SHMO a new grade of 'medical assistant' was recommended, to be of unlimited tenure and outside the training ladder, and intended for doctors who wished to work as assistants to consultants.

These highly conservative and incremental recommendations were welcomed by the Ministry and the profession, and in December 1961 regional boards were asked to set up committees to review staffing as suggested in the report. The committee established in the Leeds Region comprised seven medical and two lay members, and in addition two external assessors chosen from a panel of consultants set up by the Ministry were appointed to give guidance about the scope of the review. The review committee reported in December 1962, recommending the appointment of an additional 80 consultants and 120 registrars and house officers over a five-year period. The committee had arrived at these figures by agreeing staffing standards for each specialty, applying these standards to each hospital planning area to calculate the number of doctors required, and comparing this number with existing establishments. The committee's recommendations were intended to achieve a more even distribution of staff within the Region, and to ensure that sufficient staff were available for capital developments nearing completion, and they were approved by the Board for submission to the Ministry.

The results of other regional reviews were received by the Ministry during 1963, and the most striking feature of these reviews was the wide variation in the increases in senior staffing levels proposed by boards.[18] These increases ranged from 49 per cent in the Newcastle Region to 9 per cent in the South East Metropolitan Region, while a 20 per cent increase was proposed for the Leeds Region, somewhat below the national average of 26 per cent. Moreover, there was no correlation between boards' proposed increases and existing staffing levels. For instance, the North East Metropolitan Region demanded the second highest increase (45 per cent) even though it had the fourth highest staffing level at the time of the review; while the Sheffield Region, which had the lowest staffing level, made only the fifth highest demand for additional staff (29 per cent). Clearly, the Ministry's hope that the appointment of external assessors would 'secure a measure of uniformity between regions'[19] was not borne out. It would appear that each regional review committee adopted its own staffing standards, and that this was the main factor which explained the variations which emerged from the reviews.

A different approach was used in Scotland, where the staffing requirements of the five regional hospital boards were considered by a single committee. The significance of this committee's work lay in its attempts to 'devise for each specialty some principles of reasonable staffing in relation to work load for teaching units on the one hand and non-teaching units on the other', and then to 'consider each unit separately with such a standard in our minds without seeking merely to apply an arithmetical formula to it'. The committee claimed that: 'This attempt to relate numbers of staff to work load has not hitherto, to our knowledge, been attempted in any comprehensive way in Great Britain; and certainly it has been by far the most difficult part of our work'.[20]

The Platt working party had found the task equally difficult, and apart from suggesting guidelines for general medicine and general surgery had not formulated any standards. The attempt of the medical officers of the Leeds Board to devise staffing standards based on the estimated work load in each specialty had run up against similar problems in 1955. It will be recalled that the standards were rejected because it was felt that the number of variables which affected the work of a consultant made the application of a strict formula impossible. While recognising these problems, the Scottish committee argued that standards could be applied if adequate allowances were made for local conditions. Adopting this approach, the committee concluded that a 14 per cent increase in medical staff was needed.

This was half the increase proposed by the English and Welsh boards, whose demands were so great that they could not be met in full. Accordingly, for each specialty the Ministry took the median of boards' proposals, and, where existing staff already exceeded the median, existing staff figures were used; where boards' demands were below the median the demand figure was used; and where the demand figure was above the median, but the number of existing staff was below it, the median figure was used. As the Leeds Board's demands lay below the median the Board was granted its full demand – an extra 80 consultants. Nationally, it was planned to appoint an additional 1095 whole-time consultants over the period 1964–1968, compared with boards' demands of 1806.[21] The method used to scale down boards' demands resulted in some redistribution of consultants in favour of deprived regions, though this appeared to be more a side effect than a positive aim of national policy.

At the same time as announcing its policy on consultant expansion, the Ministry confirmed the introduction of the medical assistant grade, from 1 November 1964, and the phasing out of the SHMO and JHMO grades. Boards were asked to set up a professional committee to hear applications for regrading to consultant status from SHMOs holding allowances in recognition of their special responsibilities. Finally, the Ministry announced that revised allocations of registrar and house officer posts would not be made. Applications for additional posts in these grades would be considered as they arose, having regard to such factors as the supply of manpower and the ratio of consultants to other medical staff. This last decision exemplified the essentially passive style of manpower planning adopted by the Ministry. Among other things, the Platt reviews afforded the opportunity for a more positive approach to the problems of the medical staffing structure, with the planned expansion of the consultant grade being complemented by increases among junior doctors sufficient to bring the structure into balance, with at the same time the expansion being distributed so as to overcome geographical inequalities. But the opportunity was not taken and, as we discuss next, there continued to be problems with the staffing structure.

The hospital doctors' charter

The Platt reviews had three major effects in the Leeds Region. First, the rate of expansion of the consultant grade increased. Over the period 1953–64 an average of nine whole-time equivalent consultants was added to the Region's consultant establishment each year. As Table 4.1 shows, the rate of increase more than doubled in the next four years, with an additional 87 whole-time equivalent consultants being employed between 1964 and 1968. In the first of these years the increase was due mainly to the regrading of SHMOs with special allowances, but after that date the Platt allocations took effect and

TABLE 4.1 *Hospital medical and dental staff in the Leeds Region, 1964–9*

	Con-sultants	SHMOs Medical Assistants	Senior Registrars	Registrars	SHOs	HOs*
1964	299.3	75.0	34.2	130.8	163.7	–
1965	329.1	40.3	32.6	142.0	196.0	104.6
1966	345.6	59.7	36.3	150.0	204.5	106.6
1967	371.4	54.7	36.3	170.0	265.1	98.9
1968	386.4	57.7	34.3	160.0	301.5	92.3
1969	402.0	53.7	37.6	168.6	318.0	94.2

SOURCE *Hospital Medical and Dental Staff, 1964–1969* (each year) (London: DHSS).
All figures are whole-time equivalents, are for 30 September each year, and exclude teaching hospital.
* No figure for house officers is available for 1964.

continued into 1969. This demonstrates the importance of economic factors and the changing economic climate as an influence on medical staffing. Whereas in the early 1950s cost considerations had meant that strict controls had to be imposed on increases in the consultant grade, ten years later a more favourable, expansionary climate led these controls to be relaxed.

The second effect was a marked decline in the size and importance of the sub-consultant grade, as measured by the number of SHMOs and medical assistants in post, both absolutely and relative to the consultant grade. The medical assistant grade was never popular with junior doctors, mainly because it was outside the training ladder and was seen as being inferior to the consultant grade. At the profession's request the Ministry placed a moratorium on appointments in 1968, and although the moratorium was subsequently lifted controls continued to be exercised over the creation of new posts.

The third effect of the Platt reviews was a large expansion of the registrar and, more particularly, the senior house officer grades. As the table shows, the number of senior house officers employed in the Region almost doubled between 1964 and 1969, while the number of registrars employed rose by nearly one-third. These increases were of particular concern to junior doctors, whose career prospects were again threatened by the expansion of the training grades at a faster rate than the career grades. This concern was reflected in the formation of the Junior Hospital Doctors' Association within the British Medical Association in 1966, and in the publication of the 'Memorandum on the Current Problems of Hospital Medical Staff', which became known as the hospital doctors' 'charter', in 1967.[22]

The charter began by arguing 'Never before have hospital doctors been so disenchanted with the conditions under which they are called upon to practice', and in support of this it cited the alleged underfinancing of the NHS and the existence of outdated buildings and equipment. Behind the rhetoric lay a number of specific claims: that consultant cover in hospitals was inadequate; that there were insufficient consultant vacancies for senior registrars; and that the training needs of junior staff had been sacrificed to service requirements.

These claims raised complex issues which did not admit of simple solutions, and drew attention once again to the intrinsic difficulties of devising a satisfactory medical staffing structure for hospitals. As potential consultants, junior doctors justifiably expected time off for study and a planned training programme, together with a reasonable prospect of a consultant appointment on completion of training. On the other hand, the service needed pairs of hands to undertake the increasing volume of often routine work with which hospitals had to deal, and the number of doctors required for this purpose was not necessarily the same as the number needed to replace consultants who died or retired and to permit the steady expansion of staffing consequent on new developments. If the two were not in balance then either bottlenecks would appear in the middle grades or there would be staff shortages. Indeed, there might be bottlenecks in some specialties and shortages in others at the same time. The position was further complicated by the employment of overseas doctors, many of whom were expected to return to their own countries rather than stay on to be appointed consultants; by the emigration of British doctors; and by whether trainees chose a career in general practice or the hospital service. The charter put these issues at the top of the agenda, and marked the beginning of negotiations between the Ministry and the profession which extended over five years. Immediately though, in 1967, central controls of the registrar grade were tightened, and the effect of this in the Leeds Region can be seen in the table.

A series of reports recorded progress made in the negotiations,[23] and contributions to the debate were also made by the Royal Commission on Medical Education[24] and the Godber Report on 'The Responsibilities of the Consultant Grade'.[25] After some hesitation and internal disagreement the profession came out against a permanent sub-consultant grade in general, and the medical assistant grade in particular, as a way of solving the problems of the training grades. At the conclusion of the first round of discussions the profession's representatives had endorsed the sub-consultant grade, but at the BMA's Annual Representative Meeting in 1968 opposition, particularly from junior doctors, led the grade to be rejected. In the words of conference delegates, the grade would 'create a pool of stagnation and discontent'[26] in the profession, and it 'amounted to . . . "consultants on the cheap" '.[27] What junior doctors feared most about the grade was that it was a blind alley which offered little in the way of career prospects. The force with which these arguments were presented led senior members of the profession to acquiesce.

On the other hand, by 1972 agreement in principle had been reached on the introduction of a part-time sub-consultant grade, to

be known as the 'hospital practitioner' grade, mainly but not
exclusively for general practitioners. But the most important outcome was that the profession persuaded the Ministry to accept that
doctors would usually expect to become consultants eight years after
qualification. Once this had been decided, it was agreed that the
consultant grade should expand at the rate of 4 per cent per annum
and training grades at $2\frac{1}{2}$ per cent per annum in order to bring about
a better balance between the numbers in training for career posts and
career opportunities. At the same time provision was made for
greater medical involvement in manpower planning through a new
Central Manpower Committee and a network of regional manpower
committees. The Central Manpower Committee was given much
wider functions than its predecessor, the Advisory Committee on
Consultant Establishments, in that its role was to advise on planning
targets in the different grades and specialties and to monitor progress
in achieving these targets. It thus seemed that by 1972 a significant, if
belated, start had been made in creating the necessary machinery for
a national manpower policy, although, as the *British Medical Journal*
commented, there was 'a long haul ahead'.[28] A more positive,
interventionist approach seemed to have replaced the reactive and
passive planning style noted earlier.

One of the points which emerged during the negotiations was the
unequal distribution of hospital doctors throughout the country. As
Table 4.2 shows, in 1968 the ratio of senior medical staff per 100 000
population varied from 11.8 in the Sheffield Region to 19.1 in the
Metropolitan Regions taken together. With a ratio of 13.7 the Leeds
Region was fifth from the bottom of the regional league table. One of
the first steps taken by the Central Manpower Committee was to give
guidance on how the annual increase of 4 per cent in consultant posts
should be distributed between regions. The increases recommended
ranged from 1 per cent in the North West Metropolitan Region to 7.5
per cent in the Sheffield Region, the aim being to achieve approximate
parity in the number of consultants per head of population in each
region over a ten-year period.[29] The Leeds Region was given the fifth
highest increase – 5.1 per cent – in recognition of the leeway it had to
make up, which meant that the Board could make 30 new appointments annually compared with around 20 a year in the period
following the Platt reviews. Not only was this a further development
of the policy of achieving a more equal distribution of consultants
begun after the Platt reviews, but it was also consistent with the

TABLE 4.2   *Distribution of consultants* between regions, 1968*

England and Wales	15.2
England	15.2
Newcastle	16.7
Leeds	13.7
Sheffield	11.8
East Anglia	13.6
Metropolitan Regions (four)	19.1
Oxford	16.1
South Western	14.2
Birmingham	14.0
Manchester	13.6
Liverpool	17.3
Wessex	14.5
Wales	15.0

SOURCE   *BMJ Supplement*, 6 December 1969, p. 56. Reproduced by permission of the *British Medical Journal*.
* Consultants includes teaching hospital consultants and SHMOs with allowances.
Figures are expressed as whole-time equivalents per 100 000 population.

attempt to bring about a fairer share of financial resources between regions started in 1971.[30]

In practice not all of the additional consultant appointments were made. Between 1971 and 1975, 89 posts out of a total of 120 were filled. Four factors accounted for the shortfall.[31] First, finance was not always available to meet the revenue consequences of additional appointments. It has been estimated that in 1975 each consultant controlled resources worth £500 000,[32] and, while costs varied between areas, specialties and individuals, towards the latter part of the period 1971–5 hospital authorities found themselves unable to find the extra resources needed for new posts. Secondly, and connected with the last point, supporting facilities such as beds, theatre time and staff were sometimes lacking. Thirdly, in specialties like anaesthetics, radiology, pathology and geriatrics there were shortages of trained staff. Finally, it was not uncommon for consultants in post to oppose new appointments. As Freeman, himself a consultant, predicted in 1969, the expansion of the consultant grade was likely to be resisted by consultants themselves for three reasons: it would prejudice their income from private work; it would require facilities to be shared; and it would mean that consultants would see fewer cases of interest.[33] Events proved Freeman's prediction to be accurate.

The failure to expand the consultant grade at the expected rate was coupled with the continued expansion of the junior grades. In the Leeds Region these grades expanded by 15 per cent in 1971-1972 and 7 per cent in 1972-1973, compared with the agreed figure of $2\frac{1}{2}$ per cent. As Table 4.3 shows, the increases were greatest in the senior registrar and senior house officer grades. At the same time the number of whole-time equivalent clinical assistants employed increased from 106.4 in 1971 to 132.7 in 1973. The Region relied particularly heavily on senior house officers and clinical assistants to meet service needs as in relation to the country as a whole it had a shortage of registrars,[34] and the expansion of the registrar grade was strictly controlled by the Ministry.

TABLE 4.3   *Hospital medical and dental staff in the Leeds Region, 1969–73*

	Con-sultants	SHMO's Medical Assistants	Senior Registrars	Registrars	SHOs	HOs
1969	402.0	53.7	37.6	168.6	318.0	94.2
1970	417.1	51.3	43.0	177.0	312.0	106.0
1971	493.8*	49.2	37.0	182.0	297.0	108.0
1972	524.6	47.2	49.5	178.0	380.9	107.6
1973	544.3	34.3	54.6	183.7	434.0	98.0

SOURCE   *Hospital Medical and Dental Staff, 1969–1973* (each year) (London: DHSS).
All figures are whole-time equivalents, are for 30 September each year, and exclude teaching hospital.
* This large increase over 1970 is explained in part by a change in the method of calculating the statistics. Up to 1970 consultants known to be working maximum part-time contracts were counted as 9 sessions; after 1970 they were counted as 11 sessions.

Thus the planned differential expansion of the career and training grades in order to provide a more satisfactory career structure for hospital doctors was proving an elusive goal to implement. In fact, the apparently widening imbalance in the structure was offset in part by the employment in the junior grades of a large number of overseas doctors, many of whom were not expected to compete for career posts, or were expected to compete unsuccessfully. This factor notwithstanding, the imbalance was increasing and threatened to cause major discontent in the junior grades, yet by 1974 there was no evidence to indicate that corrective action was being taken by the Central Manpower Committee or DHSS. Indeed, all the indications were that the staffing structure was in even more of a turmoil than at any time during the previous 25 years.

Conclusion

It is difficult to escape the conclusion that the medical staffing problems experienced in the hospital service between 1948 and 1974 were not tackled as resolutely as they might have been. Responsibility for this lay with the medical profession and the Ministry of Health. As the *British Medical Journal* commented in 1972:

> The root of the hospital staffing problems really lay in the failure of successive governments and the profession to solve a deceptively simple-looking equation. How could the service requirements of the hospitals be properly met while at the same time providing adequate career training and giving established hospital doctors career and job satisfaction?[35]

Why was this equation not solved?

First, because the consultant grade did not expand at a fast enough rate, owing to lack of finance, a shortage of trained doctors in some specialties, the unwillingness of existing consultants to share facilities and private work, and the lack of supporting facilities. Secondly, because there were too many junior doctors. The Ministry failed to introduce tight enough restrictions over the senior registrar grade in the early 1950s; subsequently it allowed hospital boards to expand the registrar grade in a largely uncontrolled manner; and, when controls were introduced over the registrar grade in 1967, it permitted the senior house officer grade to expand in its place.

An underlying cause of these developments, and in the end probably the most important, was the desire of consultants to have their own supporting junior staff, and, associated with this, their antagonism to undertaking routine work themselves. As Maynard and Walker have observed:

> The pattern of medical practice in hospitals has as its core the

notion of a team of doctors led by the consultant who has ultimate clinical responsibility and who delegates tasks to the members of the team. The notion of one junior doctor for every three to five consultants is not consistent with this style of practice.[36]

And, as Freeman has argued, consultants:

feared that these proposals [to restrict junior posts] will reduce the availability of junior staff and will increase the amount of work which each consultant has to undertake (even though most are now fully committed), while at the same time making their work less professionally interesting'.[37]

Freeman also noted that consultants whose applications for extra junior staff were rejected were reluctant to see additional consultants appointed in their place. There seems no doubt that, if consultants could have been persuaded to accept a more rapid expansion of their numbers, then the imbalance in the staffing structure would have been lessened. However, the commitment of consultants to established ways of working prevented this from happening. A further contributory factor was the interest of the Ministry of Health in containing costs. Medical staffing was quite rightly seen as the key to cost containment, and although the purse strings were loosened after the Platt reviews, enabling a more rapid expansion than had been possible in the 1950s, they were drawn in again in the early 1970s with the result that some consultant posts remained unfilled.

One way around the problems of the staffing structure would have been to have increased the service contribution of the non-training grades. In fact, as we have seen, the Leeds Region did make extensive use of general practitioner clinical assistants, and the hospital practitioner grade proposals were also designed to secure greater general practitioner involvement in hospitals. However, even though the introduction of the hospital practitioner grade was agreed in principle in 1972, prolonged discussions followed on the terms and conditions of service attaching to the grade. Another policy option would have been to have actively promoted the permanent sub-consultant grade, but this was strongly resisted by junior doctors. The only remaining alternative was to go for differential expansion of the career and training grades, the policy which had evolved by the early 1970s. The power of consultants at the local level prevented this policy from being implemented: hence the more vocal expressions of discontent by junior doctors. As Elston has noted: 'By perceiving that they have not always benefited from the "partnership" that professional autonomy involves between the state and the doctors' leaders, junior doctors have attempted to enter into direct negotiation on employer-employee lines.'[38]

Thus to the main conclusion of this chapter: that the professional monopolisers are not an homogeneous group, and that one of the most significant divisions within the medical profession is between junior doctors and consultants. It was this division which caused there to be continuing problems with the medical staffing structure. After their unsuccessful attempt to intervene in the early 1950s, the corporate rationalisers at central government level contented themselves with a reactive planning role, and their failure to control junior staffing accentuated the problems of the training grades. Although the establishment of the Central Manpower Committee in 1972 was indicative of a more positive planning style, subsequent developments suggested local professionals had the power to frustrate the intentions of national policy-makers. Regional consultants continued to request additional assistance, and these requests were granted in the form of extra senior house officer posts which were outside the control of the Central Manpower Committee. There was, then, a regional backlash against the centrally-negotiated agreement, and local corporate rationalisers – that is, the Board's officers – did not intervene to prevent this; for example, by refusing to sanction new junior posts. Given their principal concern to ensure adequate medical staffing in the Region's hospitals, and the Region's shortage of registrars, it would have been surprising if they had reacted differently. Accordingly, the strategy of muddling through with the medical staffing structure continued to benefit those with power, senior members of the medical profession, although by 1974 increasing organisation among junior doctors represented a serious threat to this dominance.

5

Long-stay Services

This chapter examines and analyses in detail the development of three specific services: those for the elderly, the mentally handicapped and the mentally ill. Collectively, these are often referred to as the 'Cinderella' services, to denote their comparative neglect in the NHS. One of the consequences of this neglect has been the formation of a number of pressure groups to fight for more resources for these services. Moreover, since the late 1960s there has been a central government commitment to giving greater priority to the elderly, the mentally handicapped and the mentally ill. While policy developments in this sphere at the national level have been well documented, the local response is less well known. What, for example, was the impact of the Hospital Advisory Service (HAS) at regional and local level? How did RHBs and HMCs respond to the Ely Report? Also, since most attention has focused on developments after 1969, how did Cinderella services evolve before that date? These are some of the questions addressed in this chapter. The approach used is again analytical as well as descriptive, with an attempt being made to draw out more general points about policy processes from the specific cases discussed.

Geriatric services

Early initiatives

The wartime survey of hospital services in the Yorkshire Region found the standard of provision for the elderly and chronic sick to be far below what could reasonably be expected.[1] Voluntary hospitals were interested mainly in the acutely ill, and it was left to local authorities to provide what care they could for the chronically sick. Often this was no more than a basic level of nursing care with few attempts to undertake active treatment and rehabilitation. The hospital boards and committees which took over control in 1948 therefore faced a major task in instilling a new philosophy into the care of the aged. The task was made greater by the increasing proportion of the population which was over pensionable age. It was against this background that the Leeds Board had to plan its geriatric services.

On the advice of the Geriatrics Committee, which from 1950 to 1954 was chaired by Ronald Tunbridge, Professor of Medicine at Leeds University, the Board adopted a policy which had four interrelated aims: first, to maintain and if possible increase the number of geriatric beds in the Region; secondly, to establish admission units at general hospitals; thirdly, to appoint medical staff specialising in geriatric medicine; and, fourthly, wherever possible to plan services jointly with local health authorities.

Some of these aims proved easier to achieve than others. Thus, the number of geriatric beds available was gradually increased, with redundant infectious diseases and tuberculosis beds being converted for use by the elderly. Moreover, as early as February 1949 the Board laid down the principle that geriatric beds should not be diverted to other uses 'unless at least equally suitable alternative accommodation is available'. Board policy was to provide a minimum of 1.5 beds per thousand population in each hospital district,[2] and its desired standard was 2 beds per thousand. This contrasted with the Ministry of Health norm of 1.2 beds per thousand.[3] The difference between these figures was discussed at a conference on the care of the aged sponsored by the Board and held in June 1959. The conference was attended by over 800 people, including representatives of hospital authorities, local health authorities, general practitioners and other interested bodies. The delegates identified three reasons for not reducing the Board's standard of bed provision to conform with the Ministry's figure: first, local authority residential services were insufficiently developed, and until they were expanded extra hospital accommodation would be needed; secondly, the ageing population indicated a probable increase in the demand for beds; and, finally the comparatively recent appointment of consultant geriatricians in most areas meant that active rehabilitation and discharge policies were only just getting under way, and only when these policies were fully developed could reduced bed provision be contemplated.

Three years later the Hospital Plan showed that in providing 1.7 geriatric beds per thousand people the Leeds Region was well above the national average of 1.3. Indeed, together with the East Anglia and South Western Boards, the Leeds Board was making proportionately greater provision than any other part of the country. Yet these average standards of provision obscured considerable inter- and intra-regional inequalities. Between regions the standard varied from 1.0 to 1.7, while within the Leeds Region provision ranged from 1.1 to 2.4. The standards also took no account of the quality of the accommodation. In Halifax, for instance, there were 2.3 beds per thousand population but nearly all of these beds, like so much of the geriatric accommodation in the Region, were in a former workhouse which also contained local authority Part 3 accommodation (this was residential accommodation – old people's homes – provided under part 3 of the 1948 National Assistance Act). Replacement of the beds at St John's Hospital, Halifax, was thus one of the Board's major building priorities in the Hospital Plan.

The geriatric bed norm laid down in the Plan was 1.4 beds per thousand population, or 10 beds per thousand population aged 65 and over. This entailed a reduction of some 600 beds in the Leeds Region. In view of the pressure on existing beds, the Board was concerned at this prospect, arguing that special factors like the large-scale employment of female labour in the West Riding, the inadequate development of local authority services and poor housing conditions, justified greater than average provision of beds in the Region. The Ministry, not impressed by these arguments, asked the Board to bring its plans into conformity with national guidelines. It was the Ministry's view that the extension of local authority services foreshadowed in the Health and Welfare Plan would more than compensate for the reduction in hospital beds. Thus it was as a result of external pressure rather than internal competition for beds that the Board had to reverse its policy of increasing bed provision. But the actual impact of this was limited, and around 5000 beds continued to be available for geriatric and chronically sick patients right through the period.

There was rather slower progress in achieving the second policy aim, that of establishing an admission unit in a general hospital in each hospital district. By 1954 units existed in just over half of the districts in the Region. Where such units had not been established, it was often because of resistance from consultants in acute specialties to any reduction in 'their' beds. This was the case in York, where the Board engaged in protracted negotiations with consultants in an effort to establish a small admission unit at one of the city's two general hospitals.

The move to set up these units was often associated with the appointment of medical staff specialising in geriatric medicine, which was the third aim of Board policy. It was, in fact, as early as December 1950 that a pioneering appointment was made when Dr Hugo Droller took up post in Leeds as the Region's first consultant geriatrician. This was followed by the appointment of senior hospital medical officers at Bradford (1951), Halifax (1952) and Pontefract and Wakefield (1952), and the Region's second consultant geriatrician at Bradford in 1953. There was a steady addition to these posts in the years which followed.

In many ways the appointment of new staff was the most significant development in geriatric services because of the stimulus to improved service provision which usually followed. This was acknowledged in a report presented to the Board in 1954 which noted that in Scarborough 'the appointment of a Consultant Physician with geriatric responsibilities has given considerable impetus to the development of the service'. Reflecting on the development of geriatric medicine, Isaacs has recalled, with perhaps only a little exaggeration:

The consultant geriatrician on his appointment was usually expected to look after several hundred beds in one or more hospitals previously designated for the chronic sick. With these beds he had to provide directly for the geriatric needs of a community of perhaps a quarter of a million people, and he might also be expected to accept transfers from the local general hospitals of patients considered to be in need of long-term accommodation. He might at the outset find that his beds were occupied by patients who had long been considered as not amenable to treatment, and who had received little medical attention in the past. Geriatricians reacted to this situation in a characteristic way. Within a few weeks the wards had been transformed. The bedfast patients were all up; several had been discharged home after a very long period in hospital. Incontinence had diminished, pressure sores had healed, contractures had straightened. The ward had acquired new curtains; there were flowers at the bedsides; the plumbers had come in to see what could be done about the toilets. The visiting hours had been lengthened, and visitors, physiotherapists, occupational therapists, almoners, and voluntary workers swarmed in and out of the wards. The radiology departments and laboratories were complaining about the extra load of work thrust upon them. And the geriatrician was down at the office of the Regional Hospital Board demanding more money, more staff, and more beds.[4]

In the Leeds Region the effect of new appointments was seen in the reports from consultants and senior hospital medical officers on geriatric services in their areas, frequently containing suggestions for improvements and requests for additional equipment and facilities. While these requests were not always met in full, it was unfortunate, in view of the stimulus provided by the medical staff, that it was sometimes difficult to fill newly-created posts or posts which fell vacant. By 1959 there was an establishment of seven consultant geriatricians, yet two posts were unfilled. Likewise, two of the four senior hospital medical officer posts were unfilled. These problems, which were due to the shortage of suitably qualified candidates, continued right through the 1960s and 1970s. It was suggested that a better field of candidates might be attracted if consultant geriatricians' duties were linked with those of physicians, or even taken over by the latter. However, the Board's officers advised against such a move, arguing that the problem of amending the contracts of physicians in post and the fragmented service which was likely to result would outweigh any advantages. Commenting on this issue some years later, the Hospital Advisory Service observed that:

'joint' posts are not . . . always attractive to those wishing to specialise in geriatric medicine and sometimes a candidate is appointed who has not had training in a specialised geriatric unit. In some, usually rural, areas such joint appointments appear to work very successfully. In others there may be an incomplete commitment of the consultant appointed to the interests of the geriatric department.[5]

Experience thus tended to support the officers' advice, which was endorsed by the Board.

Local authority liaison

One of the many advantages which tended to follow from consultant appointments was the development of closer links with local authorities. The relationship between hospital and local authority services for elderly people was an issue which gave the Board considerable cause for concern. This applied in particular to those elderly people occupying hospital beds who were suitable for transfer to Part 3 accommodation. In the post-war austerity era local authorities could do little to increase this accommodation, a factor which, as we have seen, was used by the Board to justify a higher than average level of hospital provision. This issue apart, the Board's Geriatrics Committee was well aware of the need for liaison between the two services, and so it was instrumental in organising a number of regional and local meetings between HMCs, representatives of local government, and also GPs. Despite these efforts, a conference held in 1952 concluded that 'there was little or no co-ordination and that one of the crying needs of the service today was for better liaison between the various Authorities concerned'. Exactly the same conclusion was reached seven years later at the conference on the care of the aged organised by the Board, and arising out of this the Board's officers prepared a report on arrangements which existed in the Region for co-operation between the three branches of the NHS. The report noted that joint committees fully representative of hospital authorities, local health authorities and GPs existed only in Leeds and Hull. Also, although case conferences between hospital and local authority staffs took place regularly in six of the thirteen hospital districts in the Region, nowhere were three-sided case conferences held. Again, contacts with voluntary bodies were haphazard.

After discussing the report, the Board's Geriatrics Committee asked the Regional Health Services Liaison Committee to consider the establishment of joint geriatric services committees in each area along the lines of those existing in Leeds and Hull. This the Liaison Committee did in June 1960, when it emerged that the Board's enthusiasm for joint committees was not shared by the local authorities' representatives. The latter argued that while such committees had made a valuable contribution in some areas, notably Leeds, excellent liaison already existed at officer level throughout the Region. The setting up of additional committees would cause complications, particularly in those areas served by more than one authority, and bring few, if any, compensating advantages. While conscious of the need to improve liaison, the local authorities' representatives felt it was a matter on which each authority should make its own arrangements.

In putting the case for joint committees, the Board's representatives argued that there was a pressing need to ensure that patients were cared for in accommodation appropriate to their condition. The Board appreciated that there was a shortage of Part 3 accommodation, but, because of the large number of hospital patients suitable for transfer to local authorities, considered that cases should be jointly reappraised in each area. There was therefore a continuing need for discussion of common problems at the local level. Despite these arguments, the views of the local authorities prevailed, and the principle of establishing joint committees was not accepted.

This was unfortunate in view of the widely recognised success of the Leeds Joint Geriatric Services Committee in improving liaison between the hospital service, local authority services and GPs. The Committee was not a panacea, and there were many problems with geriatric services in Leeds, some of which are touched on in Chapter 6. The Committee was nevertheless effective in bringing together different interests to discuss problems of common concern. Also, at the level of day-to-day working, if not at the level of long-term planning, a number of practical improvements followed, including the secondment of a social worker to the geriatric unit and the joint assessment of cases. In considerable part these improvements were due to the pioneering work of the consultant geriatrician, Dr Hugo Droller, and the support given by the medical officer of health for the city of Leeds.[6]

The need for a joint approach to services for the elderly was underlined by the development of the Hospital Plan and the Health and Welfare Plan. In the preparation and subsequent revision of both Plans hospital authorities and local authorities had exchanged information on the services they were intending to provide, and this policy was taken a stage further in a circular issued in 1965 which stated that the provision of a single service to the elderly 'demands *joint* planning by all the responsible authorities of the provision and operation of the service'[7] (emphasis added). The circular suggested that RHBs should take the initiative in convening meetings of a group of officers of hospital and local health authorities, together with general practitioners, and with the addition of other local authority officers, like housing officials, when necessary. By sharing and assembling information these groups would 'serve as a clearing-house for considering short-term policies and administrative pro-blems as they arise in the operation of the services', and would assist in the process of reaching 'agreement on desirable priorities and long-term plans'.[8]

When the circular was considered by the Board's Geriatrics Committee, members expressed the view that 'local planning groups as such were unnecessary'. They felt that the joint discussions which were already occurring in connection with the revision of the Hospital Plan were adequate, and that what was needed was 'to put on a formal basis the consultations that already took place in most areas'. Thereafter meetings between officers continued much as before, and there is no evidence that the circular led to any greater co-ordination in the planning or delivery of services.[9] Part of the reason for this was referred to in the circular itself: the large number of different authorities involved made joint planning at one and the same time a desirable but difficult goal to achieve. A further reason was that the long-term planning of geriatric services was over-shadowed by the more immediate concern of hospital authorities to discharge elderly patients needing care rather than treatment, and the parallel concern of local authorities to secure hospital admission for the residents of their homes. It was this issue more than any other which dominated joint discussions of geriatric services and which militated against the strategic planning of those services.

The Hospital Plan and after

To return to hospital services, publication of the Hospital Plan in 1962 marked an increase in spending on geriatric services as well as services for other patient groups. However, even before publication of the Plan the Board had made some progress towards improving the quality of geriatric accommodation, most notably at Staincliffe General Hospital, Dewsbury, where a new 96-bed unit built at a cost of only £116 000 was opened in 1960. The unit comprised three L-shaped wards based on an original design by the architects and the Board's officers. In a modified form the design was adopted in later developments at St Luke's Hospital, Huddersfield, and Eastburn Hospital, near Keighley, and in part accounted for the low cost of those developments. The Staincliffe-type ward, as it became known, was also used in a scheme for the provision of additional geriatric beds at Bempton Lane Hospital, Bridlington.

Many more schemes of improvement were included in the Hospital Plan, but progress in bringing about these improvements was interrupted in 1967 when a small pressure group known as Aid for the Elderly in Government Institutions (AEGIS) alleged ill-treatment to elderly patients in psychiatric and geriatric care. These allegations were published in *Sans Everything – a Case to Answer*, which contained pseudonymous accounts of cruelty, illtreatment, neglect and unkindness to patients written by nurses and social workers at seven hospitals in six regions throughout the country.[10] To allay public concern the Minister of Health asked regional hospital boards to set up independent committees of enquiry to investigate the allegations and to consider more generally conditions at the hospitals concerned.

Two of these hospitals were in the Leeds Region: Storthes Hall Hospital, Huddersfield, which was a large, old mental illness hospital; and St James's Hospital, Leeds, which contained a large number of geriatric beds. The four-man committee of enquiry which was appointed by the Board reported in March 1968 and found that none of the allegations of cruelty or ill-treatment was justified. The only criticisms of staff made by the committee were that a nurse at St James's Hospital had sworn in the presence of patients, and that there was some evidence of inefficiency in the administration of the Hospital. The latter referred to the catering, laundry, engineering, supplies and general administrative departments, where the Committee concluded that 'certain criticisms (of a minor, or even trivial character) of the work of the Departments . . . were proved to be well-founded'. However, the committee was 'not prepared to make any findings which reflect adversely upon the work which these officers faithfully, industriously and devotedly perform each day'. Indeed, conditions generally at the two hospitals were found to be good, although the committee did recommend increases in nursing establishments and reductions in the bed complements of wards.

These findings were very much in line with those recorded by the other committees of enquiry, and summaries of the committees' reports were published in July 1968.[11] Reassuring as these reports were, they were only a response to specific cases and ignored the more general and important points of the AEGIS campaign, that hospital services for the elderly as a whole were under-staffed, under-financed, and had for too long been given low priority. The Minister of Health also ignored this point in simply requesting Boards to follow up the committees' recommendations at the hospitals investigated.

In responding to this request, the Leeds Board asked the HMCs responsible for St James's and Storthes Hall to make suggestions for improvements at the two hospitals. Subsequently the committees requested additional revenue of £86 000 and £26 000 respectively to enable more nurses to be employed. The Leeds (A) HMC also asked for an additional capital allocation of £10 000 to allow a number of minor works to be carried out. These requests were approved by the Board's Finance and General Purposes Committee but, when they came before the Board itself, it was resolved that 'the revenue expenditure involved be considered in relation to other priorities in the Region'. In the event, the Leeds Board allocated an extra £40 000 to St James's and £20 000 to Storthes Hall for 1969/1970, and so even in specific cases demands for additional revenue were met only in part.

Yet this commitment of funds did at least set a precedent. Thus, as we note below, following the Ely report the Board found £215 000 from its own allocation and resources to distribute to HMCs for expenditure on long-stay services in 1969/1970.[12] Of this sum £87 000 was spent on mental handicap services, the remainder being allocated to services for the mentally ill and elderly, and this was on top of the £60 000 already allocated to St James's and Storthes Hall. Additional sums were also made available in each of the succeeding years up to 1974. In the main these later increases came out of national increases in the NHS budget. Around half of these extra allocations was spent on staff, but recruitment continued to be a problem, and the staff shortages which remained were due not to any lack of funds but to the absence of suitable applicants for posts advertised.[13] The balance of the additional allocations was spent on items like patients' lockers and cupboards.[14] This expenditure helped to bring standards at hospitals for the elderly up to the minimum laid down by DHSS in 1972. Thus after a hesitant start the Board gradually increased its revenue commitment to these hospitals.

A much more positive commitment to geriatric services was evident in the capital programme. In reviewing the programme in March 1969, the Board decided to spend an average of 13 per cent of its capital budget in future years on geriatric services. This target was achieved in the five-year period 1969/1970 to 1973/1974, over £5 million out of a total capital expenditure of almost £40 million being spent on hospitals for the elderly. In the latter part of that period the Board benefited from the extra money allocated to the NHS by the government, much of which was spent on capital works in the long-stay sector.[15] Steady progress was therefore made in replacing old and unsatisfactory accommodation for the elderly by new building and providing more day hospitals. The only exception was Leeds, where it was decided that phase two of the redevelopment of St James's Hospital, which was a purpose-built geriatric block with comprehensive day hospital and rehabilitation facilities, should be used initially for general medical purposes. This decision, which is discussed in more detail in Chapter 6, nicely exemplifies the vulnerability of geriatric services to pressure from other specialties.

It was just this vulnerability which was referred to in a memorandum submitted to the Board in 1968 by Dr Hugo Droller, the consultant geriatrician at St James's. Although the memorandum was not addressed directly to the question of the use of phase two at St James's, it neatly encapsulated the frustrations the question had aroused amongst those most intimately involved. Droller summarised the problem as follows:

> Geriatric medicine, twenty years after its introduction, still suffers from lack of status. Although recognised by the Royal College of Physicians as one of the medical specialties which will be of steadily increasing importance, we still lack the cachet of distinction which would attract more staff, staff of higher calibre, and give us the same standing as other specialties enjoy. We are still the poor relation.

As evidence of this low status Droller instanced the fact that there was only one university chair of geriatrics in the British Isles, at Glasgow. He challenged the Board to take the lead in establishing such a chair at Leeds. At a later date the Director of the Hospital Advisory Service made a similar point in criticising medical schools· and teaching hospitals for failing to set an example, as 'centres of excellence', in developing geriatric services.[16] This criticism certainly applied to Leeds, where no beds were allocated to geriatrics in the hospitals under the control of the Board of Governors of the United Leeds Hospitals. In contrast, on the other side of the city at St

James's, Droller's work had attracted visitors from all over the world, and somewhat ironically the geriatric unit at the Hospital, even though housed in old and inadequate buildings, very justly warranted the description 'centre of excellence'.

Geriatric services were not alone in their low status. Many of the problems described above – the shortage of qualified staff, inadequate funds, and low standards of patient care – were shared by the mental handicap and mental illness services, which we discuss next. At the same time, there were a number of significant improvements in hospital services for elderly people: old buildings were replaced with new; units were established in general hospitals; and consultant and other staff were appointed, often leading to revolutionary changes in methods of care, cure and treatment. In other words, many of the deficiencies identified in the Hospital Survey were tackled with resolution. Yet with the proportion of the population over pensionable age increasing, the further development of geriatric services presented a major challenge to the NHS.

Mental handicap services

The Ely Report

Until the late 1960s mental handicap services attracted little interest and attention. These were the 'quiet backwaters'[17] of the hospital service, and only when there were allegations of ill-treatment to patients at Ely Hospital, Cardiff, in 1967, was the peace broken. It is not surprising, then, to find that the Leeds Board did not devote much time to mental handicap services. While the Mental Health Committee of the Board kept these services under review, there were no major policy developments in the first 20 years of the NHS. Small increases were made to the bed stock during the 1950s, with the result that there was some reduction in overcrowding and waiting lists in the Region's hospitals. Apart from this, the main point to note is the decision taken in 1959 to build a new hospital for the mentally handicapped at Wakefield. The intention behind this decision was to provide the Wakefield area with a comprehensive mental handicap hospital providing a full range of facilities, supported by satellite hospitals fulfilling more specialised functions, as existed in the remaining four planning areas for mental handicap services. Overall, the aim was to provide around 4400 beds, or 1.4 beds per thousand population, compared with 4000 beds in 1959 and 3400 beds in 1948. This was slightly higher than the figure of 1.3 beds per thousand population put forward as a planning norm by the Ministry of Health in the 1962 Hospital Plan. The Ministry requested the Board to bring its plans into line with this figure, arguing that greater provision of care in the community by local authorities, foreshadowed in the Mental Health Act of 1959 and outlined in the 1963 Health and Welfare Plan, would reduce the need for hospital beds. This the Board reluctantly agreed to do, and a policy for mental handicap services for the next decade and beyond was thus established.

The Ely Hospital 'scandal' marked the end of this period of slow, unobtrusive and incremental development. The Committee of Enquiry set up to investigate conditions at the Hospital reported in 1969,[18] and found that most of the allegations of ill-treatment to patients made by a nursing assistant were justified (it should be noted that the report was concerned only with the male side of the hospital). The reasons why this situation had been allowed to develop were complex, and responsibility was laid at the door of a number of individuals and agencies: nursing standards were found to be old-fashioned and custodial, and staff were inhibited in making complaints for fear of victimisation; the standard of medical care was described as 'low' and the junior hospital medical officer and physician superintendent were held responsible for this; local authority provision for the mentally handicapped was inadequate and there was a lack of co-ordination between local authority and hospital services; the Welsh Hospital Board had failed to use its powers to improve standards and oversee the work of the HMC; and the HMC itself, together with its officers and advisers, had, in the words of the report, to 'accept the principal responsibility for the shortcomings identified'.[19] The lasting impression created by the report is of the *isolation* of Ely Hospital: there was no league of friends, visits by members of the HMC were irregular and infrequent, the nursing staff were described as 'a close-knit and inward-looking community',[20] as to a lesser extent were the medical staff, whom the report felt 'should be brought into a much wider medical community'.[21] Thus, one of the most important recommendations made by the Committee was that: 'There is a clear need for some system of inspection of a hospital like Ely, which will ensure that those responsible for its management are made aware of what needs to be done to bring it up to the desired standards.'[22]

The response to Ely

Subsequent developments in mental handicap services in the Leeds Region were much influenced by the national policy response to the Ely report, and so it is appropriate to examine in a little detail the nature of that response. The Secretary of State for Social Services at the time was Richard Crossman, whose diaries contain interesting insights into the way in which the Ely issue was handled. The diaries make it clear that Crossman saw the Ely report as a personal challenge – 'I have got a cause at heart and a job I can really do'.[23] Consequently he became heavily involved in working out what should be done to prevent a recurrence of Ely and to improve standards generally at mental handicap hospitals. The first issue Crossman latched on to was the Committee of Enquiry's recommendation that a system of inspection be established. After some resistance from the medical profession and from civil servants within DHSS, Crossman succeeded in establishing the Hospital Advisory Service. It was emphasised that this was not an inspectorate, as it seemed Crossman had wanted, but rather the Secretary of State's 'eyes and ears',[24] reporting directly to him on its visits to long-stay hospitals. The second issue Crossman took up was the need to shift resources to long-stay hospitals. When he first raised this Crossman was told by the Chief Medical Officer and Permanent Secretary at DHSS that resources could not be switched from acute services to the long-stay sector without antagonising the medical profession.[25] However, at a meeting with Regional Board Chairmen on 30 April 1969 Crossman asked for reports on the implications of diverting $1\frac{1}{2}$ per cent of revenue expenditure which would have been spent on general hospital services in 1969/1970 to long-stay hospitals, with priority for the mentally handicapped. As he records in his diary: 'Here I did get into difficulties'.[26] In the Leeds Region, HMCs were strongly opposed to any diversion of funds. The York (A) HMC, for instance, which was a group containing both general and long-stay hospitals, argued that: 'first priority must be given to the building of the new District General Hospital, York . . . and there can be no question of any immediate improvement in the psychiatric and geriatric services unless additional allocations are made'. Similarly, the East Riding HMC, also a mixed group, maintained that 'any redeployment of resources would injure the deprived hospitals to a far greater extent than any benefit to the receiving hospitals could justify'. While resource reallocation was therefore rejected by HMCs, from its own reserves and allocation the Board was able to find £215 000 to distribute to HMCs, and of this £86 000 was allocated to mental handicap services.

Thus resistance from civil servants, the medical profession and hospital boards and management committees prevented any major reallocation of funds. Crossman responded in two ways: first, he asked Pauline Morris, the author of *Put Away: A Study of Mental Handicap Hospitals*, 'to give me a whole range of things which we could do to ease the position of sub-normal hospitals. These things, costing hardly any money, are what we shall have to concentrate on in the first year'.[27] The suggestions made by Morris and included in a list of improvements circulated to regional boards involved such things as making full use of leagues of friends, longer and more frequent visiting by HMC members, and arranging for the exchange of staff between hospitals. The Leeds Board commended these suggestions to the attention of HMCs and contented itself with monitoring their implementation. (This was consistent with the role of regional boards set out in Circular HM[69]59, which was a direct outcome of the Ely Report's finding that there was lack of clarity in the relationship between boards and management committees.) Crossman's other response was to earmark *additional* funds for specific services. His diary records: 'We are going to dock all regions of some £50 000 capital expenditure, and we have found another £3 million for the problem of sub-normality'.[28] Yet even here Crossman had a struggle with his civil servants, who had devised plans to spend the extra money on all long-stay services. Crossman, however, insisted on their being used only on mental handicap services, and he won the day.

Of the £3 million earmarked for these services in 1970/1971, the Leeds Board received £205 000. Additional funds were also allocated in succeeding years, and from 1972/1973 onwards these were earmarked for all long-stay services. The Board was able to find funds from its own development money to supplement these allocations, which were used for a variety of purposes, including improving food standards to bring costs up to the DHSS norm, consequential increases in catering staff, employing additional nursing staff, and providing extra GP sessions and attendances by dentists and chiropodists.

Earmarking additional funds for long-stay services was also

introduced on the capital side. In 1970/1971 DHSS withdrew £2 million from boards' planning allocations and distributed this for use on long-stay services, and in succeeding years funds over and above normal allocations were earmarked for these services. The Board's Treasurer reported that: 'The special supplement is to be used to give an additional impetus and not to be taken as justifying any reduction in the resources which would otherwise have been allocated to these services'. The additional allocations made an immediate impact on mental handicap services: in the Leeds Region capital expenditure on these services increased from £460 000 in 1969/1970 to £1.2 million in 1970/1971 and £1.17 million in 1971/1972. Although to a large extent these increases can be accounted for by the entrance of the long-planned mental handicap hospital at Wakefield into the building programme, they were also due in part to the priority the Secretary of State asked boards to give to mental handicap services. The clearest example of this was the erection of what at first were known as 'Coleshill', and later 'Crossman', units to mitigate the worst cases of overcrowding.[29] These were 30-bed prefabricated ward units with a life of 10–15 years, and eight such units were erected in the Region. In addition, two occupational therapy units of similar design were provided. Many less major improvements, like the provision of additional toilet facilities, were also carried out. Capital expenditure on mental handicap services reached a peak in the early 1970s, and thereafter declined – to £550 000 in 1972/1973 and only £290 000 in 1973/1974. This reflected the priority that was given to these services immediately after Ely and the later shift in emphasis to mental illness and geriatric services.

The Hospital Advisory Service

A stimulus to the improvement of mental handicap hospitals, apart from the earmarking of funds, came from the Hospital Advisory Service (HAS), whose first Director, Dr A. A. Baker, was appointed in November 1969. Shortly after his appointment Baker agreed an 'initial plan of operation' with DHSS. This stated that the functions of HAS were:

(i) by constructive criticism and by propagating good practices and new ideas, to help to improve the management of patient care in individual hospitals (excluding matters of individual

clinical judgement) and in the hospital service as a whole:
and
(ii) to advise the Secretary of State for Social Services about
conditions in hospitals in England and the Secretary of State
for Wales about conditions in hospitals in Wales.[30]

In 1970 Baker recruited four teams of professional advisers, each
team comprising a consultant, a senior nurse, a ward sister or charge
nurse, a hospital administrator and a social worker, usually on
secondment from the NHS. At the outset it was agreed that the teams
would concentrate on long-stay hospitals, particularly those for the
mentally handicapped. Accordingly, two teams focused on mental
handicap hospitals, the third team on mental illness hospitals and the
fourth team on geriatric and chronic sick hospitals. The teams
operated by visiting a hospital for a few days, talking with staff,
patients and HMC members, observing staff at work, and generally
entering 'into the life of the hospital as much as possible'.[31]
Following a visit a report was submitted directly to the Secretary of
State as well as RHBs and HMCs, who were then asked to inform
HAS of action taken on recommendations made.

The teams completed their visits to all mental handicap hospitals
in the Leeds Region by February 1971. However, before the HAS
visits a team of Board officers comprising a doctor, nurse, administrator and treasurer, visited these hospitals themselves between
January and March 1970 and again between August and October
1970. On both occasions the team recorded that their general
impressions were that there was no evidence of cruelty to patients,
that the standard of accommodation was good but could be
improved, that there was some overcrowding and serious staffing
shortages, and that staff were sometimes over-protective and paternal-
istic in their attitudes to patients. In between the Board's team's visits
a number of improvements were effected. At one hospital, for
example, the number of patients without personal lockers had been
reduced from 255 to 120, and all patients had personal clothing,
whereas previously 238 patients did not. This was by no means
untypical, either of the Leeds Region or of the country as a whole.[32]

Despite the steps taken by the Board during 1970, the HAS reports
identified many other improvements which were needed. Some of
these involved expenditure and the Board, after considering the
reports, allocated further revenue and capital resources to meet the

necessary cost. Others did not entail expenditure, such as the almost universal recommendation that multi-disciplinary management be introduced. Yet these were often the most difficult recommendations to implement, as they involved overcoming entrenched attitudes about the respective roles and responsibilities of different professional groups.

Like the Board's own team, the HAS was concerned at the level of overcrowding, particularly at the Region's largest mental-handicap hospital, Meanwood Park Hospital, Leeds. The Board was well aware of the problems which existed at this hospital, for in 1969, following the violent deaths of two patients, an internal enquiry had been conducted by the HMC.[33] In the first six months of 1970 the number of patients was reduced from 840 to 800 and the Board allocated an additional £70,000 to the HMC specifically for improvements to the hospital. When the HAS team visited the number of patients had been further reduced to 740, but the team identified two major outstanding problems: first, there were shortcomings in mangement, and a lack of individual responsibility and competence both at group and hospital level in more than one profession. To overcome this the formation of a management team, comprising administrators, consultants and nursing officers, was advocated. The second problem concerned the standard of nursing care, and the HAS team felt that standards and practice were lower at this hospital than at almost any other in the Region. The team therefore recommended that a small nursing team from HAS should visit the hospital to undertake a further in-depth study of the problem, and this was done during 1971. At the end of that year a report from the HMC to the Board indicated what action had been taken to improve conditions at the hospital. The number of patients in residence had fallen to 723 and overcrowding had also been reduced by the opening of two 'Crossman' ward units; a multi-disciplinary management team had been established; there had been increases in nursing and domestic staff; a variety of capital improvements had either been completed or were under way; and a start had been made on improving standards of nursing care following the special visit by the HAS nursing team. This example, which illustrates the effects of additional expenditure and the HAS on mental-handicap services, was not unusual. As Jones *et al.* comment in their study of the Region's mental handicap hospitals carried out in 1971:

It was evident that a good deal of money had recently been spent on the upgrading of physical facilities and some informants attributed this directly to the extra funds made available under the Crossman administration, and the work of the Hospital Advisory Service.[34]

Equally important as improvements to physical facilities were less tangible developments like breaking down the isolation of hospitals and changing staff attitudes. The HAS teams had some impact here, and a further stimulus to these developments was the Training Project Officer experiment launched in 1970. This was another initiative in which Richard Crossman took a personal interest. The idea behind the experiment was that each board should appoint an officer, to be known as a Training Project Officer (TPO), to bring about changes in hospitals for the mentally handicapped. The TPO role has been described as 'ambitious and ambiguous',[35] and it was primarily through practice and experience that the role became more closely defined. Pantall[36] has listed the activities which TPOs typically organised, and these included education and training by such means as regional conferences, staff training courses, and staff exchanges and visits; the dissemination of information via newsletters; and attempts to bring about organisational change – for example, by encouraging the introduction of multi-disciplinary management. Action under all of these headings was undertaken in the Leeds Region, where the TPO was assisted in her work by a Regional Working Party comprising consultants, nursing officers, a nurse tutor, hospital administrators and remedial officers. Yet the limited resources devoted to the experiment, exemplified by the fact that only one officer in each Region was employed on the project, was a major constraint on what could be achieved. Also, the expertise which was slowly built up was often dissipated as TPOs moved to other posts. For these reasons, and the vague initial conception of the experiment, TPOs tended to make only a marginal impact, even though they were potentially one of the most important innovations to follow the Ely report.

Better services for the mentally handicapped

As well as having an immediate effect on policy and service provision in the ways already described, Ely prompted a reappraisal of long-term plans for the mentally handicapped. This was reflected in the publication of the white paper, *Better Services for the Mentally Handicapped*, in 1971, which envisaged that at an unspecified date in the future hospitals would provide for a little over half of the 60 000 patients they accommodated in 1969.[37] These patients would be those who required treatment rather than care. This was a major policy change, equivalent in its way to the decision taken in 1961 to run down hospitals for the mentally ill. In response to the white paper the Leeds Board put forward plans to reduce the number of mental handicap beds in the Region from 4000 in 1970 to 2500 in the long term. Just over half of these beds were to be in existing hospitals, all of which were to be reduced in size, the remainder being provided in small new buildings close to the communities they served.

At the same time as hospital provision was reduced, there was to be an expansion of day care, and much greater provision of residential care in local authority homes and in foster homes and lodgings. The white paper asked boards to consult local authorities in preparing their development plans. However, as Jones and her colleagues comment in their study of mental handicap services in the Region:

> In 1972 and 1973 the Regional Hospital Board took the initiative in approaching Directors of Social Service, drawing their attention to the White Paper proposals and calling meetings for discussion; but the response so far has been less than enthusiastic.[38]

Although the Board's plan gave details of local authority proposals for the mentally handicapped insofar as places in adult training centres and residential homes were concerned, there had been no joint planning of services. Moreover, if past experience were any guide, then the aim of developing community care was likely to be difficult to achieve. This aim had been established in the 1963 Health and Welfare Plan which had set targets of provision for 1972. Jones and her colleagues note that:

> Local authority plans for the mentally handicapped in this Region for the period 1962/1972 were unevenly implemented. Some authorities' targets were set very low, and it was clear that this was not regarded as a priority area for development.[39]

It remained to be seen whether the Better Services white paper would meet the same fate.

Summary

The evolution of mental handicap services illustrates a number of points about the policy process. First, it shows how issues can get on to the agenda after a long period of apparently uncontroversial development. In this case the personal interest of a particularly influential individual – Richard Crossman, the Secretary of State for Social Services – was the central factor. Crossman's determination to make use of the Ely committee of enquiry's report, and to publish the report in full, ensured that mental handicap services became a matter of public debate and political response. Neither the report itself nor the events which precipitated it was sufficient to make this happen. Crossman cleverly extended the scope of concern in order to push policy in the direction he wanted.

Secondly, examining the policy response to Ely shows how Crossman's aims were modified by the other interests involved – civil servants, the medical profession, and hospital boards and committees. While he succeeded in his principal aims of establishing a system of inspection and allocating extra resources to mental handicap services, both were the result of negotiation and bargaining in a system of bureaucratic politics. It was within the decision-making interstices of DHSS and the NHS that the eventual policy was worked out. Thus the HAS was presented as an advisory service and not an inspectorate; and the shift in resources was achieved by means of earmarking extra funds instead of reallocating money within existing budgets, as Crossman had originally wanted. This meant that not only did the mentally handicapped benefit, but also that other groups and services did not lose; an important outcome in view of the anticipated reactions of the medical profession.

Thirdly, and most interestingly, the evidence from the Leeds Region indicates that the policy was implemented as intended. The Board found money from its own allocation to support developments financed by earmarked funds, and there were noticeable and measurable improvements in standards and facilities at mental handicap hospitals in the Region. There were also more intangible improvements, like the reduction in the isolation of these hospitals, and the beginning of a commitment to multi-disciplinary management.

On the negative side, however, it was by no means clear that the impetus provided by Ely would continue. We have noted how capital expenditure on mental handicap services fell from £1.2 million in 1970/1971 to £290 000 in 1973/1974. Again, the developments inspired by the HAS visits and the Board's own teams lost momentum after the initial burst of activity in 1970 and 1971. There seemed to be no means of engaging with the more intractable problems of mental handicap hospitals on a permanent basis. The HAS did not have the resources to provide a continuing service in more than exceptional cases, and the Board's project team became much less active after its first series of visits in 1970. We have noted, too, that the potentially important Training Project Officer role was never fully supported or exploited. It was not surprising, then, that later reports into conditions at other mental handicap hospitals, Farleigh and Normansfield,[40] for example, should discover problems similar to those that existed at Ely.

Also problematic was the implementation of the new plans for the mentally handicapped enshrined in the *Better Services* white paper. In particular, the divisions of responsibility between hospital and local health authorities seemed likely to make the development of community care more an aspiration than a reality. The experience of mental illness services, to which we now turn, reinforced this prognosis.

Mental illness services

Overcrowding and underspending

It would not be an exaggeration to say that, of all the difficulties facing the Board in 1948, the condition of some of the Region's mental illness hospitals gave most cause for concern. This much is clear from the early reports on these hospitals prepared by the Board's medical officers. One report described Stanley Royd Hospital, Wakefield, as follows:

> The old gaol-like buildings at Wakefield are gloomy and depressing and the galleries where many patients aimlessly spend so much of their time are deficient in natural lighting. The accommodation can best be described as austerely pre-Dickensian, falling far short of usually acceptable modern standards, and . . . there is still created in the mind of the observer an undeniable impression of

miserable discomfort and overcrowding which cannot long be tolerated under enlightened administration.

Conditions such as these were confined mainly to Stanley Royd, Storthes Hall and Menston, the three hospitals which had previously been under the control of the powerful West Riding Mental Hospitals Board, the body which ran mental illness hospitals on behalf of the county and county borough councils in the West Riding area. Elsewhere standards were higher, notably at Clifton Hospital, York, of which the Board of Control inspector commented in 1952: 'This hospital continues to be administered upon the most progressive lines, and the patients undergoing treatment enjoy the benefit of enlightened and thoughtful medical care. We have seen much to praise during our visit.' In view of what follows, it is important to note this variation in standards between hospitals at the outset. While the majority of patients were accommodated in institutions which were in urgent need of attention and improvement, others were cared for in hospitals which were among the most progressive of their day.

The most pressing overall problem in 1948 was the high level of overcrowding, estimated to be 15 per cent in the Region as a whole. A major reason for this was the large number of patients from the adjacent Newcastle and Sheffield Regions accommodated in hospitals in the Leeds Region. Another factor, peculiar to the West Riding, was that the admission block of Stanley Royd Hospital was being used for non-psychiatric cases. This was a wartime expedient which had been continued after 1945 despite undertakings that the admission block would be returned to its original use. But the hardest pressed hospital was Menston, just outside Leeds, where there was 35 per cent overcrowding. Following questions in Parliament in July 1952 the Board took belated emergency action to relieve this institution: catchment areas were revised and patients transferred to other hospitals in order to distribute the overcrowding more equally. Shortly afterwards patient 'ceilings' were introduced for each hospital to prevent a repetition of the Menston situation. These 'ceilings' could not be exceeded without the Board's approval and were intended to be a warning that overcrowding had reached unreasonable limits.

Yet there was little or no improvement in conditions at Menston as a result of this action, and the seriousness of the Hospital's problem was noted throughout the 1950s in the reports of the Board of

Control's inspectors. These reports drew attention not only to the high level of overcrowding, but also to the inadequacy of the sanitary accommodation and the shortage of medical and particularly nursing staff. These deficiencies were also highlighted in three detailed reports submitted to the Board by the Friends of Menston Hospital, an organisation representing patients' relatives. In the third of these reports, presented in July 1956, the Friends noted in particular the lack of patient activity; the poor quality of patients' food; the low standards of patients' clothing; and the adverse effects of overcrowding combined with staff shortages. In the course of their report the Friends stated:

> It is our contention that conditions at Menston *are* shocking and, whilst we have restrained our justifiable indignation in recent years, believing that by moderation we might best achieve our purpose, it may be that we have erred in our methods. (original emphasis)

The Friends met members of the Board's Mental Health Committee to discuss these points, and subsequently issued their report to the press. Although the report was couched in moderate language, it contained a number of pointed criticisms of conditions at Menston. The adverse publicity which resulted led the nursing and ancillary staff at the Hospital to call a meeting at which the Friends' action was condemned because the staff felt it would retard nurse recruitment. The Mental Health Committee of the Board responded by convening a special meeting with the Hospital Management Committee, at which the latter reiterated its strong objections to the Friends' statement. In contrast, some members of the Mental Health Committee, although not accepting the Friends' criticism of the Hospital's staff, supported the general sentiments expressed in the statement. In the event the publicity which resulted from the report had the desired effect in that it prompted the Board to allocate extra funds to Menston. Thus, an increase in the medical establishment was approved to enable the Hospital to be divided into a number of independent units, each headed by a named consultant supported by a clinical team; and discussions started on the capital improvements needed to modernise the Hospital. The improvements were initially estimated to cost £1 million, but after discussion with the Ministry of Health they were scaled down and eventually schemes to the value of

£230 000 were undertaken out of the original modernisation programme. The Ministry's view was that money should not be spent on
large, old hospitals when national policy was to build new accommodation for short-stay patients. This meant, as the HMC explained
in a report to the Board in 1965, that improvements in the standard of
patient care were still hindered by a situation in which 'the majority of
wards house 70/90 patients in five rows of beds which are often too
close together to permit even lockers between'.

In spite of this, the same report noted that a number of advances
had been made: a day care unit had been established within the
hospital grounds providing 24 places with active treatment facilities
and group therapy; industrial rehabilitation facilities had been
extended; 'living-in, working-out' had been developed, involving 30
patients; and the hospital had been divided into three self-contained
sections, headed by consultants with supporting teams, and responsible for a cross-section of wards including all types of patients.
Unfortunately, it had been impossible to link these sections with
geographical areas owing to the diversity of local authority arrangements. The catchment area of Menston included six local health
authorities, and this complicated inter-organisational co-ordination.
Again, the catchment area included a large number of family doctors,
and, while regular seminars were held at the hospital for GPs and
seven GPs had been appointed as clinical assistants, much remained
to be done to improve and extend contacts between the primary care
and hospital services.

Developments at Menston have been considered in some detail
because they illustrate the more general problems of large mental
illness hospitals during this period. A common difficulty was the
shortage of medical staff, and in a memorandum to the Mental
Health Committee in 1958, Professor G. R. Hargreaves, Nuffield
Professor of Psychiatry at Leeds University, argued that it was just
this shortage that was behind overcrowding in the Region's hospitals.
Hargreaves maintained that:

Overcrowding is only a symptom of an underlying cause, namely
'therapeutic inactivity' and a low admission and discharge rate in a
given hospital. A high admission and discharge rate and the
development of extra-mural work by the medical staff can abolish
overcrowding in a given hospital. But this can only be achieved by
a high degree of therapeutic activity affecting all patients in the

hospital and this, in turn, is only possible with adequate medical staff.

Hargreaves argued that the extent to which a hospital had adequate medical staff could be ascertained by examining the weekly doctor cost per in-patient. On that criterion the Leeds Region showed up badly – with an average cost of 4s. 2d. (21p) compared with a national average of 5s. 0d. (25p). Former county mental hospitals which had established a reputation since 1948 for their high level of therapeutic activity, high turnover and extra-mural services – Graylingwell Hospital, Chichester, and Mapperley Hospital, Nottingham, were two of the examples given – had, in most cases, a doctor cost more than double the Leeds average. Hargreaves concluded that 'in some of the psychiatric hospitals of this Region we are faced with a situation which is going from bad to worse', and he argued that this trend could be reversed only by the provision of extra medical staff.

In the light of the memorandum the Mental Health Committee decided to conduct an experiment at one psychiatric hospital in the Region to increase the medical staff establishment in order to raise the weekly doctor cost per patient to 6s. (30p). Subsequently, Stanley Royd Hospital, Wakefield, was chosen as the location for the experiment, and the medical establishment was increased from 11 to 19, including 4 extra consultants. At the same time it was decided to follow the example set at Menston by dividing the Hospital into a number of functional units each staffed by a clinical team. However, a major obstacle to achieving a high degree of therapeutic activity through increased staffing was the difficulty in finding suitably qualified candidates for new posts. This was especially true in the Region's largest mental hospitals – Menston, Stanley Royd, and Storthes Hall – all of which contained over 2,000 patients, a high proportion of these being chronic cases. In 1959 the medical establishment at Storthes Hall was increased from 12 to 25 in line with increases at the other two hospitals, but the possibilities of filling this were remote because, even within the original establishment, three posts were vacant. As the Board recognised, the solution to this problem, insofar as the solution was within the Board's control, lay in making these huge psychiatric hospitals more attractive to work in by reducing their size and spending money on improvements and modernisation.

The Mental Health Act and the Hospital Plan

These aims were consistent with the thinking behind the 1959 Mental Health Act and the Hospital Plan. The 1959 Act was a landmark in the development of mental health services, and at the time of its promulgation it was viewed as the legislative expression of the more humane and enlightened attitude towards mental disorder which had developed in the 1950s. The provisions of the Act, which closely followed the recommendations of the Royal Commission on Mental Illness and Mental Deficiency,[41] had two main aims: first, to ensure that as many patients as possible were treated on a voluntary basis, with compulsory detention being used only when absolutely essential; and, secondly, to shift the emphasis from institutional care to community care. The need to move patients out of hospital and into the community was reaffirmed in 1961 when the Minister of Health, Enoch Powell, made his famous 'water-tower' speech at the annual conference of the National Association for Mental Health. Powell told the conference that in 15 years' time only half the existing number of mental illness beds would be required. This implied 'nothing less than the elimination of by far the greater part of this country's mental hospitals as they stand today'.[42] The Minister's announcement was later amplified by a circular and by publication of the calculations on which the announcement was based.[43] These calculations, carried out by Tooth and Brooke, two statisticians at the General Register Office, were based on an extrapolation of trends established between 1954 and 1959. Since these were unusual years in mental health services, in that the use of drugs led to the introduction of new methods and patterns of treatment, a number of commentators questioned whether the planned rundown of hospitals could and should take place. The circular outlining the new policy was slightly more cautious than the Minister had been in his speech, indicating that it appeared probable that over 16 years the number of beds allocated to mental illness could be reduced from 150 000 (or 3.5 beds per thousand population) to 80 000 (or 1.8 beds per thousand population). The circular emphasised that these could not be regarded as 'exact predictions'. Nevertheless:

> It seems beyond any reasonable doubt that they do give a clear indication of future trends, and that over the next 15 to 20 years there will be a large and progressive decline in the need for beds for

the treatment of mental illness, which may amount to something like 50 per cent.[44]

Regional hospital boards were asked to plan their services on this assumption. The need was to develop out-patient and day-patient facilities, and to increase the number of acute units at general hospitals. Provision would also need to be made for medium- and long-stay patients, but the Ministry felt it 'unlikely that any more large old-style mental hospitals will be built'. A wide ranging review of existing mental hospitals was called for, the aim being to prepare ten-year programmes for inclusion in the Hospital Plan, and 'to ensure that no more money than is necessary for short term use is spent on the upgrading or reconditioning of mental hospitals which in ten or fifteen years' time are not going to be required for some different purpose'.[45]

The publication of the Hospital Plan and the Health and Welfare Plan marked a further stage in the development of the new policy. The latter indicated that local authorities were planning to increase the number of centres for the mentally ill from 23 in 1962 to 103 in 1972, and to increase the number of places in hostels for the mentally ill from 340 to 4812 in the same period. The Hospital Plan showed that RHBs were planning to provide some 92 000 beds for mental illness by 1975, compared with almost 152 000 beds in 1960. In the Hospital Plan the Ministry pointed out that the estimated bed requirement for 1975 took 'no account of any contributions from expanded community mental health services'.[46] Although the expansion of these services might be expected to have 'a considerable effect on the hospital provision that will need to be made for the mentally ill in the future',[47] this was not the key to the success of the policy. Rather, the Ministry's estimates were based on such factors as advances in therapeutic methods and the provision of more extensive and accessible out-patient, day-patient and in-patient facilities, which had already led to a fall in the in-patient population.

These proposals were received with not a little scepticism in the Leeds Region. Board members and officers had reservations on two counts: first, that the reduction in beds would take place as quickly as planned; and, secondly, that local authority services would expand at the expected rate. To clarify the first point, the Mental Health Committee took the lead in getting the Board to commission a census of the patients in its psychiatric hospitals in an attempt to assess more accurately the future need for hospital provision. The census, which covered all 9762 patients in the Region's psychiatric hospitals in 1963, provided a wealth of valuable information. It showed, for example, that 54.3 per cent of patients were visited monthly or more often; 14.2 per cent were visited only once or twice a year; and 31.5 per cent never received visitors. The authors of the census paid special attention to long-stay patients, who accounted for 70.8 per cent of the in-patient population. They estimated that over half of the patients in this category would still be alive in 1975. Moreover, a number of factors combined to make the discharge of the long-stay patient extremely difficult. The authors therefore felt that the Ministry was being over-optimistic in stating that none of the existing long-stay patients in hospitals would remain after 16 years. Indeed, after reviewing likely developments in community care and treatment methods, the authors argued that between 9000 and 10 000 beds would be needed in 1975, compared with 5840 as estimated in the Hospital Plan. The authors concluded:

> It is, of course, always possible to discharge patients and empty beds by administrative decisions; but it seems clear from the survey that, in the absence of some major and favourable change in the situation, this could only be done at the cost of much hardship to patients and their families.[48]

As far as the development of local authority services was concerned, joint discussions between the Board, HMCs and local authorities took place during 1959 and 1960, following which local authorities submitted revised proposals to the Ministry of Health for community services to be provided under Section 28 of the NHS Act, 1946. Reporting on these discussions, the Board's officers noted that, while 'good progress' had been made, there were a number of obstacles to providing comprehensive psychiatric services. The most important obstacle was the modesty of local authorities' proposals, and this was confirmed by the 1963 Health and Welfare Plan. It seemed that there was a greater commitment to community care within central government than local government. Also, as critics pointed out, the concept of community care advocated by the Ministry of Health was extremely vague, most often being interpreted negatively as care not provided in hospital.

Yet a practical example of an attempt to establish a comprehensive mental health service existed in the Leeds Region in York.[49] This had started in 1953 and was influenced by experience of running a similar service in Portsmouth. Working under the aegis of a joint committee, comprising representatives of the city council and the York 'A' and Tadcaster HMC, the service revolved around a mental health centre which provided care and after-care, out-patient facilities, and a social club for former patients. The centre was also used for weekly case conferences which served as a focus for the staff involved. These staff included psychiatric social workers, mental welfare officers and psychiatrists. In 1956 the Board sanctioned the appointment of a senior hospital medical officer to be employed for 6/11ths of his time by the hospital authority and 5/11ths of his time by the local authority. This officer had general oversight of the service. Other facilities provided were a day hospital and an industrial rehabilitation unit. There were also two hostels, one being a pre-discharge unit in the grounds of Bootham Park Hospital, the other being a local authority unit. The service as a whole was run and financed jointly by the HMC and local authority, and, according to Lindsey, it 'won wide commendation'[50] as an example of how a comprehensive mental health service could be organised. The only other comparable initiative in the Region was at Hull, where the Board and the local authority co-operated in establishing a day centre providing a variety of services including electrical treatment, occupational therapy, and group and individual psychotherapy. In other areas it appeared that the commitment to developing services in the community and to joint working between hospital authorities and local authorities was much weaker, and this did not augur well for the policy of expanding community care.

But what effect did this policy have on hospital services? The main effect in the Leeds Region was to reduce considerably the proportion of capital expenditure allocated to hospitals for the mentally ill and handicapped. In the early years of the NHS around 20 per cent of the Region's capital budget was spent on these hospitals, and this was very much in line with the Ministry of Health's recommended minimum figure.[51] However, in order to give greater priority to this sector, in 1953 the Ministry announced that it was going to set aside money specifically to provide additional beds for the mentally ill and handicapped. This was what became known as the 'mental million' programme, and allocations totalling £207 000 were made to the Leeds Region between 1954 and 1957. As a consequence, the proportion of capital expenditure going on mental illness and handicap hospitals reached a peak of 37 per cent in 1955/1956. Thereafter it declined, falling to 10.7 per cent in both 1962/1963 and 1963/1964.[52] The cause of this was the reorientation of policy away from hospitals and towards the community, and within the hospital service away from separate provision for the mentally ill and towards the integration of psychiatry within general hospitals. The impact of this policy on Menston Hospital has already been described. Likewise, only essential capital expenditure was incurred at Storthes Hall Hospital, near Huddersfield. Stanley Royd Hospital, Wakefield, fared somewhat better, and a five stage modernisation programme was carried out in the 1960s. Yet overall both the Board and the Ministry sought to spend as little on the large, old mental illness hospitals in the Region as was compatible with maintaining minimum standards of care.

The main capital investment in the mental illness sector therefore went into units outside those hospitals. However, the provision of psychiatric units in general hospitals proceeded slowly in the Leeds Region. A report from the Board's officer in 1956 noted that: 'The extension of psychiatric accommodation in general hospitals has never been a popular suggestion in this Region and proposals in this direction have not been seriously discussed'. In 1960 only two such units were in operation, at St James's Hospital, Leeds, and Kingston General Hospital, Hull. The Leeds facilities were described by the Board of Control's inspectors in their 1959 report as being 'on rather a primitive scale', while the Hull unit comprised only 16 beds. In the next 14 years only two more units were provided, at the new Airedale General Hospital and at Halifax General Hospital. In addition, new psychiatric units with day places were provided at St Luke's Hospital, Huddersfield, which apart from mental illness beds contained mainly geriatric beds and a limited number of acute beds, and at Lynfield Mount Hospital, Bradford, which also contained long-stay psychiatric beds. In the case of these last two units, the aim was to provide a comprehensive service to a specified area. This was a reflection of the views of a number of members of the Mental Health Committee who were not convinced of the case for acute units in general hospitals, fearing that these would 'cream off' acute patients and turn the large old hospitals into dumping grounds for the chronically sick. Instead, a policy of developing smaller hospitals or units to provide a total service – 'consuming their own smoke' – and staffed by nurses and doctors from existing hospitals was pursued.

This policy came under review in the late 1960s when the Board was informed of a change in DHSS thinking. In future, boards were asked to provide not just acute psychiatric facilities at DGHs, but a comprehensive service with supporting day-hospital and community facilities. These changes were incorporated in Circular HM(71)97, 'Hospital services for the mentally ill', published in December 1971. In place of the previous guideline of 1.8 beds per thousand population, this circular stated that a population of 60 000 should be served by a 30-bed unit (0.5 beds/1000 population), together with day-patient (0.65 places/1000 population) and out-patient services, supported and supplemented by various community services provided by local authorities. The need for the joint planning, development and operation of services was thus once again emphasised, and central to the concept of a comprehensive integrated hospital and community service was the 'therapeutic team', comprising medical staff, nurses, occupational therapists and social workers, each team serving a population of 60 000.

Perhaps wisely, no time-scale was given for the implementation of the new policy, and in submitting its plan to DHSS in 1972 the Leeds Board stated that its proposals were 'essentially of a long-term nature, much of the development being unlikely to take place until after 1980'. Although there had been a steady decline in the number of mental illness beds available in the Region – from 11 450 in 1960 to 8300 in 1973 – it seemed unlikely that the Hospital Plan target of 5840 beds for 1975 would be met. The reason for this was the continued presence in hospitals of long-stay patients first admitted in the 1950s or earlier. Also, local authority services for the mentally ill had not developed as anticipated, and so movement out of hospital was delayed. On both counts the census of psychiatric patients in the Region's hospitals carried out in 1963 was proved correct.

Secure units

The run down of mental illness hospitals and the development of community care are the two most discussed consequences of the Mental Health Act and the Hospital Plan. Two rather neglected consequences were the effects on patients treated under secure conditions and the abolition of the Board of Control. As far as the first point is concerned, throughout the 1950s there was a steady reduction in the number of patients in locked wards, and this 'open door' policy was given a further stimulus by the liberal provisions of the 1959 Act. As a result, in 1962 only 768 patients out of a total of some 9500 were in locked accommodation in the Leeds Region, and it was considered that only 542 of these patients really needed to be in such accommodation.[53] To an increasing extent the Special Hospitals – Broadmoor, Moss Side and Rampton – took responsibility for patients needing treatment under secure conditions, and ordinary mental hospitals accepted fewer patients of this type.

This development assisted in creating more enlightened attitudes towards mental illness and mental hospitals, for, as Clare has commented: 'The wholesale unlocking of wards was seen as a tremendous step forward and as the single most effective factor in altering the image of psychiatric care over the past quarter of a century'.[54] Yet Clare goes on to note some less beneficial consequences: patients came to be categorised as either dangerous or safe, and the needs of patients who, though normally safe, were potentially dangerous were overlooked. The Ministry of Health was aware of this problem and appointed a Working Party to investigate. The Working Party reported in 1961 and emphasised the need to provide secure accommodation for patients who did not require the facilities of the Special Hospitals. The Ministry commended the Working Party's recommendations to Regional Boards in a circular which asked Boards to review their security arrangements.[55] The review carried out in the Leeds Region revealed that all but one of the patients in locked wards were in four large hospitals. Professional opinion was in favour of the designation of these hospitals as providing secure units for the Region, and against the establishment of a single Regional Secure Unit because of the adverse effect it was claimed this would have on the hospital where it was situated. Although the Ministry approved this policy it was not implemented because the HMCs concerned objected, believing that the establishment of designated secure units would mean that the hospitals with such units would be asked to accept cases from the already overcrowded Special Hospitals, and that this was not acceptable. The issue was therefore reconsidered, and the Board accepted the views of its HMCs in deciding not to designate secure units. The Board informed the Ministry that patients requiring secure accommodation as laid down in the circular should be confined to the Special Hospitals.

When the question arose again in 1972 the Board canvassed the views of HMCs and found there was still opposition to the creation of secure units in existing hospitals. This opposition came from both the members of HMCs and hospital doctors. For example, it was reported to the Mental Health Committee that: 'The East Riding Hospital Management Committee . . . supports the view of the Division of Psychiatry that such a unit should not be established in the area but should be attached to any new prison which might be built'. Again, the Wakefield HMC was only prepared to accept a unit if it were provided in a new purpose-built block. This response was not peculiar to the Leeds Region, for, as the Butler Committee later discovered, despite the Ministry's advice not a single secure unit was established in ordinary psychiatric hospitals.[56] As Clare has noted, as well as putting undue pressure on the Special Hospitals, this neglect had the effect of placing many psychiatrically-ill people in the prisons and led to an increase in the number of potentially violent patients in the community.[57] This was undoubtedly one of the failures of the 'open door' policy.

The Hospital Advisory Service

The abolition of the Board of Control left a gap in the system of monitoring conditions at mental illness and mental handicap hospitals. Prior to 1959 the Board's reports had provided a useful outside view of standards in the Region's hospitals, but after that date it was left to members and officers of hospital authorities to fill the gap that had been created. The only exception occurred in 1963 when mental nursing officers from the Ministry visited and reported on conditions at mental illness hospitals in the Region. At the end of a detailed report the officers stated: 'Although we were impressed by the progress made we were still more struck by the vast amount still to be done'. Members of the Mental Health Committee welcomed the report and informed the Ministry that they were in favour of annual visits. A similar view was expressed in a paper published in 1964 by Arthur Bowen, a consultant psychiatrist in the Region, who from 1958 to 1961 had acted as consultant adviser in psychiatry to the Board.[58] In his paper Bowen argued for the establishment of teams of psychiatrists to undertake repeated surveys of mental illness hospitals.

These calls for some form of visits, surveys or inspection received recognition in the formation of the Hospital Advisory Service in 1969 following the Ely report. The HAS team which visited mental illness hospitals adopted a different approach from the mental handicap teams. Instead of attempting to visit all hospitals, at the outset the mental illness team spent two weeks in one or two large hospitals in each region in order 'to obtain a general impression of the service across the country as a whole'.[59] Only when this had been completed and a second mental illness team set up in 1971 was coverage extended to all mental illness hospitals. The Leeds Board therefore received the first HAS report on a mental illness hospital in the Region in December 1970, and reports on the remaining hospitals followed in 1973.

The first report identified both good and bad features of the hospital visited, Broadgate Hospital, Beverley. On the positive side, the programme of ward upgrading which had recently been carried out was found to be good, and the HAS team felt that the organisation of the disturbed wards might provide a model for similar wards in other hospitals. On the negative side, the most worrying feature was the way medical work was organised. The medical staff committee had been moribund for some years, and the medical superintendent relied on informal discussions with his consultant colleagues. Of the three consultants concerned with adult psychiatry – A, B and C – consultant C worked at twice the pace of consultant A and consultant A at twice the pace of consultant B. The HAS team recommended that a fourth consultant should be appointed, and that DHSS should be asked to advise on medical organisation at the hospital. Both of these recommendations were implemented.

The team also recommended that regular meetings should take place between the medical superintendent, the hospital secretary and the principal nursing officer. These meetings had in fact started shortly before the HAS visit, but were given additional impetus by the recommendation. Concern was also expressed at the lack of attention given to long-stay patients and the failure of the consultants to involve themselves in various rehabilitation activities organised on the initiative of the nursing staff. These problems stemmed from the poor organisation of medical work, and the team recommended that, when this was reviewed and a fourth consultant appointed, the consultants' time should be adjusted to allow for work with long-stay patients and for involvement in a rehabilitation working party which it was recommended should co-ordinate rehabilitation activities. As far as the Board was concerned, one of the team's principal recommendations was that the sanitary annexes, which were described as 'appalling', should be upgraded, and on receiving this advice the Board allocated £60 000 to allow the necessary improvements to be carried out.

Although this report indicated that all might not be well in the Region's hospitals for the mentally ill, it was not until a year later on publication of the report of the Committee of Enquiry into Whittingham Hospital,[60] which was situated in the Manchester Region, that the Board gave those hospitals the same attention as had been given to mental handicap hospitals. Whittingham was a 2000-bed hospital which had many parallels with Ely. Ill-treatment of patients was confined to one part of the Hospital; the medical and nursing staff were working in isolation; and the Regional Board and HMC had failed in their management task. Despite its many similarities with the Ely report, the Whittingham report did not foreshadow another series of DHSS initiatives to improve conditions at long-stay hospitals. As the Secretary of State explained in his foreword, the reason for this was that action was already being taken 'on a wide front'.[61] An example was the advice DHSS issued on minimum standards in hospitals for the mentally ill. These standards covered all types of staff, food costs, ward space, clothing, rehabilitation and recreational facilities. The Department stressed that the standards were minimum not optimum, and the target date for their achievement was set as the end of 1974, except for domestic staff where the date was March 1973. To help Boards meet these targets the Department earmarked additional revenue funds for all long-stay services, not just mental handicap services as previously, from 1972/1973 onwards. Boards were asked to supplement these earmarked funds from their own development money.

This had been the practice of the Leeds Board since the Ely report, and as a result there had been some improvement in conditions at mental illness hospitals. Unfortunately, progress was often hampered by the difficulty in recruiting staff, especially at the large and more isolated hospitals. The money was available, but the applicants were not. Statistics for 1973 showed that seven of the eight mental illness hospitals in the Region with 200 or more beds were below one or more of the minimum standards set by DHSS. The most common deficiency in the Region and the country as a whole was that patients did not have personal cupboards. Following close behind was the continuing shortage of domestic staff.[62] Hence, even though extra money was allocated it still proved difficult to remedy such deficiencies.

If the Whittingham report had only a limited impact on DHSS, it had a major effect in the Leeds Region. With its strong criticism of the Manchester RHB, the report motivated officers and members of the Leeds Board to take action to ensure that conditions such as were found at Whittingham did not obtain in the Region. Thus three Board members accompanied by senior officers visited the Region's six largest mental illness hospitals during March and May 1972. The members did not inspect the hospitals or see patients but confined themselves to discussions with members and staff of the hospitals and HMCs. The main points made by the members in their report to the Board were that there was a substantial number of patients who could leave hospital if alternative accommodation were available; that within hospitals there was a need to develop multi-disciplinary systems of management; that there were shortages of medical and nursing staff; and that long-stay patients were rarely visited by medical staff. With regard to the last point, the report commented:

> The introduction of the Cogwheel machinery has not (so far, at any rate) contributed to a solution of this particularly intractable problem, since individual consultants take differing views about the importance of regular visits to long-stay patients.

A further impression gained by the members was 'the lack of overall authority, direction and responsibility' in the hospitals visited.

After considering the report, the Board asked HMCs to keep under review the arrangements made for medical visits to and assessment of long-stay patients, and to approach local authorities regarding the number of patients who could be discharged from hospital if local authority accommodation were provided. The Board also employed management consultants to advise on the introduction of multi-disciplinary management at one hospital. Despite these actions, many of the comments made by the members were repeated in the HAS reports on the Region's hospitals and units for the mentally ill received during 1973, giving an indication that the pace of change in these hospitals was often very slow. While each of the HAS reports contained observations and recommendations peculiar to the hospital concerned, they also included a number of recurring themes. These were that multi-disciplinary management should be introduced where it did not exist and strengthened where it did; that the rehabilitation of patients should be given greater priority; that staff should visit other hospitals to broaden their experiences and see examples of good practice in operation; that each psychiatric hospital and unit should formulate a policy and priorities document; and that medical work should be better co-ordinated. In almost all hospitals visited, the HAS team commented on the individualism of consultants, their failure to make full use of other staff in therapeutic teams, the need to establish such teams and associate them with a specific part of a hospital's catchment area, and the problems created by wards to which several consultants admitted patients. These problems were so acute at one hospital visited that a consultant and a nurse from the Service paid a return visit to give more detailed advice and assistance to the staff.

As most of the reports were not received until the end of 1973, it fell mainly to the Yorkshire Regional Health Authority to take action on the recommendations made. Hence, at this juncture it is appropriate to attempt an initial assessment of the effect of the HAS.[63] The first and most obvious effect was that hospitals for the mentally ill and mentally handicapped received more attention and more resources. The programme of visits by members and officers and the allocation of additional revenue and capital both before and after HAS visits were testimony to this. Secondly, the Service performed a useful function in disseminating ideas and information, and this benefited members of HAS teams as well as the staff of the hospitals visited. Thirdly, in reporting directly to the Secretary of State the Service was able to keep policy-makers at the highest level informed of conditions at long-stay hospitals. As the Secretary of State's 'eyes and ears', HAS helped to ensure that long-stay services continued to receive priority. Fourthly, in many cases hospital staff welcomed the opportunity offered by HAS team visits to discuss their work with fellow professionals, to explain the initiatives they were making, and to hear of developments in other parts of the country. Fifthly, the Service took on the important role of change agent, questioning established practices and encouraging innovations.

However, HAS was not universally welcomed, and team visits and reports sometimes occasioned resistance and even hostility. In the Leeds Region this was particularly noticeable following the visits to mental illness hospitals, which gave rise to many adverse comments from the staff of the hospitals and HMCs. At a special meeting with the Director of HAS held on 16 November 1973 the Board argued that staff morale had been lowered by the HAS team's visit because the team gave advice to senior hospital staff in the presence of junior staff; advice was often offered without any indication being given of how barriers to its fulfilment might be overcome; advice was given on the basis of line management rather than consensus management, which appeared inconsistent with the team's advocacy of consensus, multi-disciplinary management; and errors of fact made during discussions were repeated in written reports despite correction. One of the Service's strongest critics in the Leeds Region, a consultant psychiatrist, felt that HAS had done more harm than good for two reasons: first, it tended to operate as enquiry by gossip and rumour; and, secondly, a team would visit a hospital with 'its brief sticking out of its ears'. In other words, teams seemed to have the same solution for the problems of every hospital, but since these problems varied the HAS lost credibility.

For these reasons advice given was sometimes ignored or rejected, and this was not restricted to the Leeds Region. For example, the Report of the Committee of Enquiry into St Augustine's Hospital, Canterbury, noted that a 1971 report from HAS 'was on the whole tolerated rather than welcomed, and that some points were resented'. Moreover, 'no action was subsequently taken on important parts of the report'.[64] In its annual report for 1975, HAS observed that a disturbing feature of committee of enquiry reports was that 'a number of previous relevant Hospital Advisory Service recommendations have not been implemented'.[65] One reason why recommendations were not always implemented was the weakness in the system of follow-up reports. The Service was not informed of action taken on all items of advice given, and in the 1972 annual report the Director complained of 'insufficient feedback with which to monitor . . . progress'.[66] In an attempt to overcome this, the Health Advisory Service, created in 1976 out of the Hospital Advisory Service, was given the power to follow up reports, and it had direct access to Ministers if not satisfied.

Another factor limiting the effectiveness of HAS was that other than in a few cases the Service did not make repeat visits to hospitals. Connected with this point, and taking the analysis a stage further, it can be suggested that a basic flaw in the conception of HAS was the notion that changes could be brought about as a result of relatively short visits. The Service was only too conscious of this, and the experiment in which a special HAS nursing team spent some time at one of the hospitals for the mentally handicapped in the Leeds Region to help staff improve standards of nursing care was an attempt to overcome this problem. Similarly, in 1973 a consultant psychiatrist and a nurse administrator made special visits to 10 mental illness hospitals throughout the country, including one in the Leeds Region. In these special visits members of HAS adopted 'an enabling and catalytic role'[67] assisting hospital staff solve problems they had themselves identified. These experiments were an explicit recognition that, while normal HAS team visits might be successful in securing immediate and visible improvements to patients' amenities and surroundings, the more intractable problems concerned with staff attitudes, professional autonomy and lack of communication could only be tackled over a longer period by a heavier investment of resources. Unfortunately, this in-depth work could not be extended precisely because of the limited resources available to HAS. Indeed, after operating with four teams since its inception, HAS was reduced to two teams in November 1973 'because of the need to ease the pressure of work for hospital service management in the period around the reorganisation of the National Health Service'.[68] The need for detailed work in individual hospitals where particularly complex problems were identified therefore remained unmet, other than in exceptional cases.

Conclusions

The development of mental illness services is instructive not just for what it tells us about these services but also for the light it sheds on the processes of policy-making and implementation. At Board level what is interesting is the way in which the Mental Health Committee continually fought for more resources for the mental illness sector. As early as 1952 the Committee's Chairman made a plea at a Board meeting for the converted EMS hospital at Fulford, York, to be used as a mental hospital in order to relieve overcrowding. The Board's rejection of this plea illustrates the struggle faced by members of the

Committee. As one of the Committee's longest serving members recalled:

> The Mental Health Committee was a large one, with a most active Chairman, and a great deal of pressure was applied by the Committee to secure a larger share of the capital moneys available, because of the sorry state of many of the hospitals, but it was always an uphill fight, and it did not in fact achieve a great deal of success until special moneys became available . . . The claims of the more exciting departments within the Hospital service usually won the day when the battle for capital requirements was being considered.

This underlines the more general point that services for the mentally ill, and also, it should be added, the mentally handicapped and the elderly, tend to receive low priority because they lack status in relation to the 'more exciting' specialties. Donald Gould makes the point in the following way:

> Physicians and surgeons concerned with the diagnosis and treatment of acute conditions (like heart surgeons, chest physicians, neurologists and gynaecologists) are held in higher esteem than doctors who deal with chronic but possbly equally distressing and disabling afflictions, such as the degenerative diseases of old age, or mental illness, or affection of the skin, or V.D. It is the experts in the 'five-star' specialties who become the leaders of the profession, and who wield the greatest influence with politicians and health authorities, and . . . it is they who obtain the lion's share of available funds. The lowlier specialists and practitioners, and the patients they serve, have to make do with what's left over.[69]

These values also tend to be transmitted during and perpetuated by medical education, producing the kinds of shortages in medical manpower in the Cinderella services noted in this chapter.

The Mental Health Committee clearly faced a difficult task, and wherever possible the Committee made use of outside reports, like those from the Board of Control, and Friends of Menston Hospital, and the Ministry's mental nursing officers, to bolster its claims, occasionally with some success. These reports were an important means of getting an issue on to the agenda as, in a national context, the Whittingham report later showed. What the Whittingham report also demonstrated was that the objective conditions of mental illness hospitals, as measured by factors like overcrowding levels, were not as significant as committee of enquiry reports and press and public interest in bringing about a policy response. Objectively, conditions at mental illness hospitals were far worse in the 1950s than in the 1960s, yet with the exception of the mental million programme it was not until the late 1960s that there was a significant response in terms of the setting of minimum standards, the earmarking of funds and the introduction of HAS.

There was, however, sometimes a gap between national policy response and local action, a 'failure' in the implementation process. This was illustrated by the non-implementation of the policy of providing secure units. Although the Secretary of State at a later date earmarked funds to tempt health authorities to build these units, he had no power of direction with which to overcome local public and professional resistance to secure accommodation, and at the time of writing no regional secure units are in operation. Again, the national policy of providing psychiatric units in general hospitals was not pursued vigorously in the Leeds Region because of reservations held by a number of members of the Mental Health Committee. The Committee evolved its own policy of developing some acute units at general hospitals, while at the same time establishing small units providing a comprehensive service, separate from both general hospitals and the large old psychiatric hospitals. The 1963 census of psychiatric patients, whose conclusions contradicted the Tooth-Brooke projections, was used to justify this policy. Thus the Board, in following the Mental Health Committee's lead, exercised a real policy-making role in the mental illness sphere, and did not simply apply national policy in the Region.

The policy of providing community care was also unevenly implemented, and this was partly because of lack of enthusiasm by local authorities and partly because of cutbacks in expenditure by central government. As DHSS acknowledged in 1975:

By and large the non-hospital community resources are still minimal, though where facilities have been developed they have in general proved successful. The failure, for which central government as much as local government is responsible, to develop anything approaching adequate social services is perhaps the greatest disappointment of the last 15 years.[70]

There was also very little joint activity by hospital authorities and local authorities, the main exception in the Leeds Region being in York, where a comprehensive mental health service had been in existence since 1953. Kathleen Jones has argued that successful examples of hospital and local authority co-ordination in mental health in Britain were:

> based on a double accident: an administrative situation where hospital and local authority boundaries were roughly co-terminous, or at least easily assimilable, and an accident of personality that provided them with psychiatrists willing to reach out into the community and to experiment with a community based service.[71]

These conditions certainly obtained in York, and also in the Leeds geriatric services, where we noted earlier that there was good co-ordination of services. The complexities of liaison between hospital and local authorities are considered more fully in Chapter 7.

6

Hospital Services in Leeds

One of the concessions Aneurin Bevan made to the medical profession in drawing up his plans for the National Health Service was to allow teaching hospitals to be administered separately by boards of governors, combining the function of regional hospital boards and hospital management committees, and in direct contact with the Ministry. It was hoped that these hospitals would become centres of excellence and by their example encourage the adoption of the best clinical practices in each region. They would also, of course, provide research and teaching facilities for university medical schools. In November 1947 the Minister announced that the Leeds teaching hospitals would comprise a small number of hospitals centred around the Leeds General Infirmary (commonly known as the LGI). Collectively these became known as the United Leeds Hospitals.

In this chapter a number of issues connected with the development of hospital services in Leeds between 1948 and 1974 are examined. As in previous chapters, the aim is not just to give an account of what happened, but also to analyse why it happened. This means asking questions like who was involved in policy-making, how were problems defined, what was the policy response, and so on. Leeds has been singled out for special comment and treatment because services in the city occupied a good deal of the Board's time and attention, and because of the complexity of relations between different agencies and interests. Apart from the Regional Board and the Board of Governors of the United Leeds Hospitals, other agencies involved with hospitals in Leeds were the University, which was concerned to ensure that there were adequate teaching and research facilities for its staff and students; the Leeds 'A' and 'B' Hospital Management

Committees, which were responsible for administering regional hospitals in the city; and, on occasion, the local health authority and general practitioners.

Just as important as the number of different agencies was the multiplicity of interests, particularly medical interests. Cities with medical schools seem to attract strong and unusual medical personalities, and Leeds was no exception. The interplay between these interests and agencies is examined in relation to the problem of acute admissions to the Leeds hospitals; the evolution of geriatric services; and the development of paediatric services. It should be noted that what follows is not an attempt to give a comprehensive account of the. development of hospital services in Leeds. Rather, the more limited goal of describing and analysing a few of the main issues concerning Leeds which came before the Board is pursued. In order to understand the full complexities of these issues it is necessary first of all to sketch in some of the context within which they were played out.

The key factor to appreciate is the rivalry which has always existed between the city's two main hospitals: the LGI, a former voluntary hospital with a distinguished history; and St James's, a former municipal hospital administered by the Leeds 'A' HMC on behalf of the Regional Board. As the only teaching hospital in the Region, the LGI stood somewhat aloof from other hospitals, proudly maintaining its independence through the Board of Governors. St James's, in contrast, was the brash young challenger, young that is in terms of its development as an acute hospital rather than the age of its buildings, which were a legacy from the days when it had been used, and indeed built, as a workhouse. Before 5 July 1948 Leeds City Council had gone some way towards building up St James's into a modern acute hospital, and one of the most important steps, symbolically as well as materially, was the appointment of the first whole-time consultant surgeon and physician at the hospital in 1948. Prior to that year the beds at St James's had been under the control of consultants at the LGI, who were resistant to the claim for independence being staked on 'the other side of the city'. The development of St James's was accelerated after 1948, and the old rivalry between the two hospitals continued to have a considerable bearing on policy-making.

Before going on to examine specific issues, it may be helpful to mention briefly one or two general points about developments between 1948 and 1974. Overlapping membership and joint committees were the main formal means of collaboration between the

Regional Board and the Board of Governors. Apart from the Standing Joint Advisory Committee, which also included University representatives, the most significant joint committee was the working party appointed in 1959 to review services and make proposals for developments, in preparation for the Hospital Plan. This recommended that acute services should be provided in three hospitals: a new teaching hospital to replace the LGI; a reconstructed St James's with a reduced bed complement; and a new regional hospital. Although approved, these proposals were overtaken by plans to increase the size of the new LGI, caused in part by the planned increase in the number of medical students. The consequence was that the proposal to build a new regional hospital was abandoned, and a revised development plan for St James's was worked out.

The increase in the intake of medical students also affected St James's, which had always played a part in medical education. Even before 1948 there were facilities at the Hospital for the clinical teaching of obstetrics, and in 1949 a professorial medical unit was established. In 1950, 50 medical and surgical beds were allocated for teaching purposes, and in 1964 the teaching of geriatrics commenced. Shortly afterwards, the University approached the Board to ask for extra teaching facilities to be made available at St James's, as the United Leeds Hospitals were already working to full teaching capacity. This the Board agreed to do, and as a first step St James's took 20 students a year from 1965 to allow the medical school's annual intake to be increased to 80. Plans were then made for St James's to accept a further 40 students from 1973. At the same time the University Grants Committee agreed to finance the construction of a clinical sciences block at the Hospital.

In view of the increasing involvement of St James's in medical teaching, the Board asked the Secretary of State to designate the Hospital a university hospital under the terms of the Health Service and Public Health Act, 1968. The Board's case was supported by the University and accepted by the Secretary of State, and from October 1970 the hospitals under the control of the Leeds (A) HMC were designated as a university hospital and the name of the group was changed to the Leeds (St James's) University Group. Subsequently, additional funds were allocated to the group to enable standards to be brought up to those expected of a university hospital. Apart from the material impact of this, in terms of improved facilities and the like, the designation was of great symbolic importance in view of the long-standing competition between St James's and the LGI. Significantly, the Board of Governors neither supported nor opposed the Board's case to the Secretary of State. The minutes of the Standing Joint Advisory Committee record that the Board of Governors' representatives 'indicated that they did not consider it incumbent on the Board of Governors to comment on the proposals, and Sir Donald Kaberry (Chairman of the Board of Governors) reserved his position'. The old rivalry between the LGI and St James's was thus again in evidence, and various aspects of this are illustrated in the cases which follow.

Acute admissions

The issue which best illustrates that rivalry is that of acute hospital admissions in Leeds. For reasons which have never been fully understood, the Leeds hospitals experience a higher rate of acute medical admissions than comparable cities. These admissions go to either the LGI or St James's, and in 1948 the latter had approximately twice the number of medical beds as the former. While both hospitals were under considerable strain, it was the LGI, because of its smaller number of beds, which suffered most. Hence, throughout the 1950s the Board of Governors, under pressure from consultants at the LGI, made repeated representations to the Regional Board to the effect that St James's should take the strain off the LGI by accepting a higher proportion of acute admissions.

The views of the consultants were expressed in a memorandum prepared by Professors Hartfall and Tunbridge and Dr Towers, which was considered by the Regional Board in February 1957. The memorandum stated that the high number of emergency admissions to the LGI – in particular, medical cases during the winter months – meant that the Infirmary was not performing its proper function as a teaching hospital. The consultants argued that there was a shortage of beds for suitable research cases, and that medical firms were being deprived of interesting teaching material. They suggested therefore that St James's should take more acute cases, thus enabling the LGI to select its patients from the waiting list.

Although having sympathy for these views, the Regional Board was constrained in its ability to help by the poor facilities for emergency admissions at St James's. Also, there was a strict limit to the number of acute surgical admissions the Hospital could accept as it had only three operating theatres. Nevertheless, the Board did assist in two ways: first, from 1 January 1955 a system of alternate day admissions to the two Hospitals was instituted for emergency orthopaedic cases; and this was extended to acute medical cases in November 1957 following a two-month experiment. However, the severe winter of 1957 caused the emergency admission rate in Leeds to rise by 30 per cent and, while St James's took a higher proportion of acute medical cases, the LGI gained little relief from the alternate day admissions system.

Consequently, the Board of Governors requested further assistance, and in reporting to the Regional Board the Senior Administrative Medical Officer (SAMO) raised a proposal which had been rejected some years earlier: that a bed bureau should be established to co-ordinate admissions. In making this recommendation the SAMO was supported by the Board of Governors, but opposed by members of the Regional Board and the Leeds (A) HMC, who feared that the bureau might be used to channel the less attractive cases away from the LGI, thereby turning St James's into a 'dumping ground'. The proposal was therefore rejected, and instead, in an attempt to reduce the pressure on the Leeds hospitals, the Regional Board decided to write to GPs asking them to send patients whose residence was outside the city to the nearest general hospital.

This did no more than scratch the surface of the problem, which remained as intractable as ever. As a result, in the summer of 1959 the Board of Governors, frustrated at what it interpreted as non-co-operation on the part of the Regional Board, unilaterally decided to end its 'ever-open door' policy. It announced that from October not more than 50 per cent of the LGI's general medical and surgical beds were to be used for acute cases. This came as a complete surprise to the Regional Board, which was forced to take urgent action. In association with the chairmen of the standing committees, the Board's officers made contingency plans which were later approved by the General Purposes Committee: 110 medical beds were earmarked for use in hospitals near Leeds to cope with the expected increase in demand; and a bed bureau was set up at St James's to deal with cases diverted from the LGI and to co-ordinate admissions generally. Despite these measures, St James's was put under extreme pressure, but somewhat ironically the LGI found that it lacked sufficient surgical cases for teaching purposes.

The system of alternate day admissions to the two hospitals was therefore re-introduced in November 1960, with support from the bed bureau at St James's. This system operated throughout the 1960s, and other hospitals in and around Leeds continued to give assistance. Yet the basic problem remained as serious as ever, especially in the winter months when the rate of acute medical admissions markedly increased. During these months it became common practice for waiting list admissions to St James's to be suspended and for surgical wards to be diverted for use by medical cases, with a consequent lengthening of waiting lists. The bed bureau provided a valuable service to GPs, but it never functioned satisfactorily because a large number of patients presented themselves at casualty departments without warning, and because the bureau lacked teeth. It was described by interviewees as having 'responsibility without authority' as it could not force other hospitals to accept patients which St James's was unable to admit.

Again, the alternate day admissions system did not always operate smoothly, and a complaint voiced by those working at St James's was that the LGI would often 'shut up shop early' on its 'take' days. Nevertheless, the system continued to operate with support from the bed bureau, though in practice both hospitals admitted acute cases every day for several months of the year. Many meetings were held between the two Boards, the Leeds HMCs, the local health authority, consultants and GPs in search of a solution. Some help was given in 1970, when it was agreed that peripheral areas of the city should look to hospitals outside Leeds for emergency treatments, and again in 1971 when the first phase of the redevelopment of St James's, which included new accident and emergency and out-patient departments, was opened. While these facilities enabled St James's to perform its function as an accident and emergency centre more effectively, a solution to the problem of acute admissions remained elusive right up to 1974.

Apart from illustrating the continuing rivalry between St James's and the LGI, and the conflict between service and teaching needs, the most interesting aspect of the acute admissions issue is the way in which the problem was defined. With the benefit of hindsight, a number of those most closely involved argued that the problem was not simply one of making adequate arrangements for acute admissions, and therefore responding in terms of alternate day admission systems, bed bureaus and the like. Rather *it was a problem of providing an effective geriatric service*, both within and outside hospital, and that this had been only imperfectly perceived at the time. In other words, the high rate of acute medical admissions in the winter months, which was at the root of the problem, caused beds to be blocked by elderly patients, or 'stickers' as they were called. The solution to this problem lay partly in providing adequate community support to prevent medical–social admissions and to facilitate early discharge; and partly in providing an active geriatric service at both major hospitals. Neither condition, it was argued, was met. Although there was a good geriatric service at St James's, the accommodation and facilities there were much in need of improvement, while the LGI, like many teaching hospitals, had no designated geriatric beds before 1974. And only in the mid 1960s was the city's sole geriatrician – Dr Droller – given an honorary appointment at the teaching hospital. Working with little support, Droller could make only limited progress in unblocking beds by discharging patients to other hospitals. One of those interviewed during the research argued that an act of 'enlightened self-interest' by the main body of medical staff in support of geriatric services was needed, and that this was not forthcoming.

What is interesting, then, is the way in which one particular definition of the problem came to predominate. Not surprisingly, this was the definition of certain powerful medical interests at the University and the teaching hospital. In response to 'their' beds being blocked, they asserted the primacy of teaching cases and research material and sought means of achieving this. The problem was not defined as how to provide a service which would actively cater for the needs of patients who were blocking beds, but rather as how to pass these patients on elsewhere, preferably to St James's. The issue of how to provide an effective geriatric service did not appear on the agenda. And, of course, the dominant definition had the advantage that it did not make a claim on resources at the LGI and the University.

In seeking to explain this it is not necessary to invoke conspiracy theories. The explanation in part is that the policy-making strategy used did not encourage a comprehensive and detailed analysis of the acute admissions problem, which might have revealed that an inadequate geriatric service was the cause. Instead, a strategy of disjointed incrementalism was pursued,[1] with small changes to the existing pattern of services occurring – not always in the same direction. The other part of the explanation is that some sections of the medical profession were more powerful than others, a conclusion reinforced by the next case we consider.

Geriatric services

The rebuilding of St James's Hospital on its existing site was a complex undertaking. Essentially it involved a phased development programme, during which some patients had to be transferred on a temporary basis to other parts of the hospital or to hospitals elsewhere in the city. As part of this programme, it was planned to move geriatric patients out of what was known as the North Hospital into Phase 2 of development, which was a 200-bed geriatric block containing day hospital, out-patient and rehabilitation facilities. The accommodation vacated would then be used for general medical cases occupying beds in another part of the Hospital, E block, which was to be demolished to make way for Phase 3. This at least was the plan up to 1968.

It was at that time that the redevelopment of St James's was reviewed, and a decision was taken to use Phase 2 not as a geriatric block but as a general medical block with teaching facilities. Part of the reason for this was the unsuitability of the North Hospital for general medicine because the beds there were separated from essential supporting facilities. For service reasons, then, it was decided to leave the geriatric beds in the North Hospital, and to transfer the medical beds to Phase 2.

A second, and in some eyes a more important, reason for the change for policy was the increasing role of St James's in medical education. The success of the Board in making a case to the Secretary of State for St James's to be designated a university hospital has already been described. Intrinsic to that case was the need to have available good facilities in order to attract a professor of medicine to work at the Hospital. In the words of one of those centrally involved, Phase 2 was 'a perfect teaching block' and in order to 'tempt' a professor to St James's a decision was taken – against the wishes of the city's only geriatrician – to convert the block for use for general medicine with the addition of a professorial unit.

This illustrates again very clearly the weakness of geriatricians in the battle for scarce resources. The odds were stacked heavily in favour of acute services, with the majority of medical staff and key local administrators emphasising the important *service* reasons behind the change of use. At the same time, the Board, the HMC and the University were anxious for St James's to be designated a university hospital. In the face of the these powerful interests, geriatric services lost out and had to be content with accommodation considered unsuitable for acute services.

One of the interesting things about this issue is that in carrying out the research two competing interpretations of what happened were encountered. One interpretation stressed the service reasons for the change, and argued that the case being made for university hospital status was of secondary importance. The other interpretation reversed this emphasis, maintaining that the key factor was the need to provide good teaching accommodation and to attract a professor of medicine. To complicate matters, an administrator at Board level indicated in an interview that service reasons were given as the explanation for the change of use as a *post hoc* justification for what was in fact a decision which resulted from the greater power of acute medical interests.

This lesson was not lost on those involved in geriatric services. In 1971 the HMC put forward a proposal to exchange 270 geriatric beds at St James's for a similar number of acute beds at Chapel Allerton Hospital, which had formerly been a Ministry of Pensions hospital. The proposal was designed to achieve a further centralisation of acute services at St James's and to enable the Hospital to develop more rapidly as a teaching hospital. A particularly important factor which lay behind the proposal was the inadequacy of operating theatres at Chapel Allerton, the expense involved in carrying out improvements, and the need to move neurosurgery into St James's in order that it could be close to the new accident and emergency facilities included in Phase 1 of the Hospital's redevelopment. A detailed case along these lines was put by the HMC to the Board.

However, the geriatricians (there were by this time two consultant geriatricians in Leeds) opposed the proposal, arguing that Chapel Allerton Hospital was unsuitable and that geriatric services should remain in St James's. In support of their argument they enlisted the help of local MPs, and appealed also to the Secretary of State, who happened to be a Leeds MP. This proved effective, and the Secretary of State asked the Board to reconsider the plans taking account of DHSS policy that half the geriatric beds in an area should be in a district general hospital. Subsequently, a much less fundamental bed reallocation was implemented. The view of the original proposers of the centralisation plan was that the failure to carry through the plan served only to store up difficulties until a later date.

Thus, by extending the scope of conflict the geriatricians successfully resisted the attempt to move their beds out of St James's. This is an excellent illustration of Schattschneider's discussion of the contagiousness of conflict, and in particular his point that the outcome of any conflict is determined by the extent to which the central participants involve outsiders. Schattschneider maintains that: 'Private conflicts are taken into the public arena precisely because someone wants to make certain that the power ratio among the private interests most immediately involved shall not prevail'.[2] This fits the above case very well, and the geriatricians' strategy of politicising the conflict was clearly an attempt to overcome the inequalities of power between themselves and the medical interests which had been demonstrated by the change of use of Phase 2. Rather more complicated issues are illustrated by the development of paediatric services, which we discuss next.

Paediatric services

The city of Leeds has never had a separate children's hospital. Up to 1948, children's hospital services were provided in the LGI and St James's Hospital. These services were generally agreed to be unsatisfactory. Thus the wartime Hospital Survey noted 'the inadequacy of children's accommodation in the hospitals at Leeds is one of the most outstanding deficiencies'[3] in the Region, a judgement reiterated in the initial review of services carried out by the Board's medical advisory committees. The problem was partly one of lack of beds, and partly one of sub-standard accommodation. To overcome these deficiencies the Board set its long term aim as being the establishment of a 200-bed children's unit at Seacroft Hospital, formerly an infectious diseases hospital, to replace the accommodation at St James's and to supplement the beds at the LGI. As a start, 60 children's beds were made available at Seacroft in 1951.

Although bringing about some improvement, the inadequacy of these arrangements was forcibly pointed out to the Board in 1952 in a memorandum prepared by Professor W. S. Craig, professor of paediatrics at Leeds University. Craig maintained that paediatric services in Leeds did not 'bear comparison with those in other University towns', and he blamed this on 'the lack of any clearly defined hospital paediatrics policy on the part of the Regional Board'. The main defect, he said, was that paediatric beds were scattered among three hospitals, and he urged a policy of pooling and concentration. Further, the absence of satisfactory facilities meant that teaching and research activities were severely impaired. Craig recommended that a 'master plan' should be drawn up to secure co-ordination, and that the task of formulating this plan should be given to a standing joint paediatric committee representing administrative, nursing, surgical and medical staff.

The Board gave careful consideration to Craig's memorandum, and set up a special committee to investigate the points he had made. The outcome was that the policy of developing services at Seacroft and the LGI was reaffirmed. However, lack of funds prevented the early implementation of this policy, and in 1957 the University, under pressure from Professor Craig, again approached the Board with a view to accelerating the Seacroft developments. A meeting was arranged with Ministry of Health officials, and at the meeting these officials indicated a change of Ministry policy in favour of integrating paediatric services in general hospitals, not their separate development as was being proposed in the case of Seacroft. As a result the Board reconsidered its plans and decided, as the first and most urgent step, to concentrate medical paediatric accommodation in a 96-bed unit at St James's, at the same time providing temporary out-patient facilities.

These revised plans suffered a setback early in 1959 when the Board invited the Board of Governors and the University to form a joint working party to study hospital developments in Leeds as a whole. While planning of the paediatric unit at St James's continued, the Board stipulated that tenders for the scheme should not be sought until future policy had been considered in the light of the report of the working party, which was not completed until November 1960. In line with previously agreed policy, the working party recommended that paediatric services should be concentrated at the LGI and St James's, but it advised that the proposal to provide a 96-bed unit at St James's by the remodelling of an existing block should be reconsidered. The Board subsequently decided to build a completely new children's block at the Hospital, and this scheme was included in the Hospital Plan of 1962. Subsequently, there were a number of changes in the St James's redevelopment plan, with the paediatric unit of 150 beds eventually being incorporated into Phase 3 of developments. In

1967 the starting date of Phase 3 was brought forward to 1971 at the request of the University, which was seeking the early provision of additional and improved children's hospital facilities in order to attract a successor to Professor Craig, who was soon to retire. At about the same time as Phase 3 was due to start it was hoped that work would also commence on the new LGI, which was to include 100 children's beds.

While these plans were being laid for the future, the children's beds at St James's were transferred to Seacroft Hospital in 1966 so that the block which contained these beds could be demolished to make way for Phase 1 of developments at St James's. Thus, with the exception of a small number of surgical beds, all children's beds at regional hospitals in Leeds, and therefore the bulk of the children's beds in the city, became concentrated at Seacroft. Although it was intended to transfer these beds back to St James's on completion of Phase 3 of developments at that Hospital, Seacroft had effectively become the children's hospital for Leeds, albeit as a temporary measure only. The wheel had turned full circle then, as the Board's policy in the early 1950s had been to develop Seacroft in just this way.

A new professor of paediatrics, R. W. Smithells, was appointed in 1968, and soon after taking up post Smithells expressed his dissatisfaction with the development plans, arguing the advantages of a single children's medical centre of 300 beds at either the LGI or St James's. The Board rejected this proposal on the grounds that it would further delay the planned improvements. Having failed to convince the Board of his case, Smithells went to DHSS and, although he lost the case for a single centre, he persuaded the Department to increase by 50 the number of children's beds to be provided at the LGI. Subsequently, Smithells and some of his consultant colleagues raised objections to the paediatric unit planned for St James's, maintaining that it should include operating theatre and x-ray facilities. In the face of these objections the Board decided to replan the unit as part of Phase 4 of developments at St James's. As this phase was not due to be completed until the mid 1980s, the Board agreed to a number of improvements at Seacroft Hospital being included in the capital programme.

The future of Seacroft as the main regional children's hospital for Leeds was thereby assured for at least fifteen years. Later cuts in expenditure on hospital building, affecting both the new LGI and the development of St James's beyond Phase 3, appeared likely to cause this period to be extended. It is therefore almost certain that the paediatric policy of the 1950s – to provide a unit of 100 beds at the LGI and a 200-bed unit at Seacroft – will obtain in the foreseeable future, and it must remain doubtful whether paediatric accommodation will ever be fully integrated into the general hospitals in Leeds.

The history of this issue illustrates some of the complexities of hospital planning. Above all, perhaps, it exemplifies the gap between intention and action, between policy-making and policy implementation. Throughout the period under review there was an identifiable policy, albeit a changing policy, on children's hospital services in Leeds. Why, then, was this policy not implemented? At least part of the answer is that the large number of different interests involved – the Board itself, clinicians, the University, the Board of Governors, and the Ministry – made it difficult to secure agreement on what should be done. While there was unanimity on the nature of the problem – too few beds in poor accommodation in too many hospitals – there were differences of opinion on what the policy response should be. In particular, there was a division between the clinicians, whose favoured policy was the provision of a single paediatric unit, and the Board, which argued for two units. This had two effects: first, it slowed down the decision-making process by requiring lengthy consultation through such mechanisms as special committees and joint working parties; and, secondly, some interests had an effective veto over development proposals, thus causing occasional policy review and change. The clearest example of the latter was the opposition of clinicians to the plans for a new paediatric unit at St James's Hospital, leading to the revision of these plans in the early 1970s.

This is an illustration of the more general rule that, in policy systems where there are many different interests and where power is not concentrated in an individual or group, it is easier to prevent change than to achieve it. Successful policy promotion in such systems is dependent on the winning of a coalition of support by an active individual or interest. In a case such as this, it might be expected that clinical interests, specifically those of the Professor of Paediatrics and his colleagues, would provide sufficient impetus to overcome stalemate. This did not happen for the greater part of the period under review. Professor Craig refused to become involved in the Board's medical advisory machinery, shunning repeated overtures from his colleagues that he join them in putting pressure on the Board through the committee system.[4] To use a military metaphor, Craig was more inclined to wage guerilla warfare by memoranda than fight a set battle at the committee table. There seems little doubt that the development and implementation of an effective policy was hindered as a result. In contrast, Craig's successor, Professor Smithells, became heavily involved both within and outside the committee system in pressing for improved services. As we have seen, this had the effect of causing the children's unit at St James's to be deferred from Phase 3 to Phase 4, and, together with reductions in public expenditure, it meant the delay for many years of the implementation of the desired policy. In summary, this case is an example of 'non-decision-making', and in particular of the way in which 'demands for change in the existing allocation of benefits and privileges in the community can be . . . maimed or destroyed in the decision-implementing stage of the policy processes'.[5]

Conclusions

While each of the cases just described has its own peculiarities and illustrates different aspects of the policy process, there are a number of common and predominant themes. The first is the sheer organisational complexity of policy-making in Leeds, particularly as a result of the separate administration of the teaching hospital. But what difference would an integrated hospital service have made? It can be argued that if the United Leeds Hospitals had been administered by an HMC under the overall control of the Regional Board then the difficulties encountered would not have been overcome. Instead, they would have been perpetuated in an alternative form, with one HMC championing the interests of St James's and another the interests of the LGI, leaving the Regional Board in the position of deciding how far and in what way to intervene. On the other hand, a single HMC for the whole of Leeds might have been more effective in securing agreement and action on the sorts of problems we have discussed.

However, this organisational reform would not have eradicated the political complexities of policy-making in Leeds, represented by the variety of different interests, particularly medical interests, in the city. In analysing the interplay between these interests a number of tools from the policy analysis literature have been used: Braybrooke and Lindblom's discussion of disjointed incrementalism; Bachrach and Baratz's work on non-decision-making; and Schattschneider's consideration of the contagiousness of conflict. Indeed, in relation to Schattschneider's analysis, one of the interesting issues to emerge from this chapter is the changing nature of the alliances that were forged: the University, for example, pressed the Regional Board for action on acute admissions and paediatric services, but gave its support to the proposal that St James's be designated a university hospital; and the intervention of local MPs and the Secretary of State on the side of the geriatricians in their opposition to the centralisation of acute services was as decisive as their non-involvement in the decision to change the use of Phase 2 of St James's.

All of this suggests a highly plural system with different interests winning out over different issues. But was this really the case? Closer inspection of the data reveals that, while decision-making processes approximated to the bureaucratic politics model outlined by Allison,[6] with compromise, conflict and bargaining being the dominant features, the balance of power was weighed heavily in favour of teaching interests and acute services. These were the interests and services which were predominant in 1948, and they maintained their position because, as we have argued, the multiplicity of organisations and interests in Leeds tended to favour the *status quo*. To use Alford's terminology,[7] the corporate rationalisers did not seriously challenge the professional monopolisers, and the community population was most notable by its absence. Alford's analysis needs to be qualified by noting that among professional monopolisers some groups were much stronger than others, and, to simplify only a little, the development of services in Leeds is very largely the story of how these stronger groups sought to maintain and enhance their positions.

7

Liaison with Other Agencies

In Chapter 5 we discussed a number of aspects of liaison between hospital authorities and local authorities, in the context of services for the elderly, the mentally ill and the mentally handicapped. In this chapter we examine liaison more generally, considering relationships between the Board and executive councils, as well as relationships between the Board and local authorities. We shall again be asking: Who was involved in these relationships? What approach to policy making was used? And so on. At the end of the chapter we seek to assess what experience in the Leeds Region has to tell us about inter-organisational relationships in the NHS. To begin with, though, it may be helpful to recapitulate the functions of executive councils and local health authorities.

Executive councils were set up under the 1946 National Health Service Act to administer the contracts of family practitioners – that is, GPs, dentists, opticians and pharmacists. Councils were nominated by local practitioners, local authorities, and the Minister of Health, and they took over the work of the former Insurance Committees. Their functions involved 'mainly record-keeping and wage dispensing',[1] though they also performed the important task of hearing patients' complaints. Alongside each council were a number of statutory professional advisory committees, including the local medical committee whose members usually comprised local BMA leaders.

Local health authorities were responsible for a range of services, including maternity and child welfare services, midwives, health visitors, vaccination and immunisation, home helps, ambulances, home nurses, health centres and health education. Local authorities had, of course, a long history of providing health services, including hospitals. The effect of the 1946 Act was to transfer hospitals to regional hospital boards and hospital management committees; to make the provision of some services mandatory rather than permissive; and to add other services to those already being provided. Local authorities were also required to provide various welfare services for those in need of care and attention under Part 3 of the National Assistance Act of 1948. As far as the NHS was concerned, the most significant of these services was residential accommodation for the elderly (commonly known as Part 3 accommodation). It is the relationship between the Leeds Board and local health authorities in the Region that we discuss first.

Liaison with local health authorities

The early years

Officers and members of the Board were in contact with officers and members of local health authorities on an informal basis from the very beginning of the Board's existence in order to ensure that the transfer of functions which took place on 5 July 1948 occurred smoothly. As early as May 1948 a conference was held in Leeds to discuss joint consultant appointments and the respective roles of hospital almoners and social workers, and delegates referred these and other matters of common concern to the Board's main medical advisory committee, the Specialist Services Advisory Committee, and local authority medical officers of health, who organised themselves into a Liaison Committee. The two committees paid particular attention to the organisation of tuberculosis services, since tuberculosis was not only the most pressing problem facing the NHS in 1948, but also required close co-operation between hospital and local authority services if it were to be tackled effectively. Following intensive discussions at officer level and a further conference of members, it was agreed that:

social, preventive and after-care work in tuberculosis being inseparable from the clinical work of the chest physician, he should act as Consultant Adviser to the Local Health Authority under the administrative direction of the Medical Officer of Health.

This arrangement worked well, and the Board was reimbursed by local authorities for the time its chest physicians spent carrying out preventive duties at chest clinics. But there was less agreement on the part to be played by health visitors and social workers, and because practice and opinion varied throughout the Region it was left to each local authority to work out its own policy.

Services for the elderly also required close co-operation, and in an effort to achieve this the Board took the initiative in organising a series of local and regional meetings between hospital management committees, local authorities and GPs. One of the major problems identified at these meetings was the difficulty of arranging for the interchange of patients between hospitals and Part 3 accommodation. Another problem, as expressed in the report of the regional conference on geriatric services held in April 1952, was that 'there was little or no co-ordination and that one of the crying needs of the service today was for better liaison between the various Authorities concerned'. A notable exception to this existed in Leeds, where in 1951 the two hospital management committees, executive council and local authority formed a joint geriatric services committee. A local authority social worker was seconded to the geriatric unit, and visited and reported on applicants for hospital admission. On the basis of these visits and reports from GPs, the consultant geriatrician then decided priorities for admission. In his turn, the geriatrician acted as an adviser to the local authority, not only on health and welfare services but also in relation to the housing needs of the elderly. But the Leeds arrangements were one of the few examples of good collaborative practice in the Region. Elsewhere much remained to be done.

At regional level overlapping membership between the Board and local authorities was one of the principal channels of liaison, and local authority members comprised about a quarter of total Board membership. Another channel was the Medical Officers of Health Liaison Committee, which met monthly with the Board's medical officers. This link was strengthened by the appointment of medical officers of health to the Board's medical advisory committees. The Liaison Committee was the main source of advice to the Board on local health authority matters, and recommendations from the Committee were forwarded to the Specialist Services Advisory Committee. One example was the proposal made in October 1949 that a standard ambulance admission form be used throughout the Region.

Significantly, this proposal drew an objection from the West Riding County Council, which informed the Board that 'it was somewhat disturbing to find that matters within the province of a Council Committee were being dealt with by an *ad hoc* meeting of medical officers'. The Council added that it seemed 'the Board was under the impression that the medical officers spoke with the authority of their respective Councils'. As this was not necessarily the case, the Council suggested the formation of an advisory committee of elected members as well as officers.

The Board accepted the Council's suggestion and, in 1951, a Regional Liaison Committee was set up 'to consider and advise the Regional Hospital Board and the Local Health Authorities on matters of mutual interest'. The Committee comprised four Board members, two members of each county council and one member of each county borough council in the Region. A year later the Central Health Services Council published an important report on co-operation between hospital, local authority and general practitioner services, emphasising the need to secure co-operation at local as well as regional level.[2] A local liaison committee covering all health services did in fact exist in Hull, and the question of whether this example should be copied in the rest of the Region was debated in November 1952 at a conference between the Board, HMCs, local authorities and GPs. However, by 56 votes to 27 the delegates decided that, while co-operation was desirable, 'this Conference is of opinion that such co-operation can best be achieved by the goodwill of the authorities affected and by local and informal arrangements, rather than by the setting up of special consultative committees for the purpose'.

This confirmed the Guillebaud Committee's observation that there was 'a general reluctance to add to the proliferation of committees already existing in the Service'.[3] Objections to local liaison committees were raised again in 1959, when the Board suggested that such committees should be set up to co-ordinate services for the elderly, and in 1965, when the Ministry of Health made a similar suggestion.[4] It seemed that local health authorities were resistant to any proposals that committees should be established uniformly throughout the Region, instead of being left to local discretion.

The Guillebaud Committee believed that more time was needed for co-operation between agencies to develop, and it identified three levels at which co-ordination was needed: first, at the central level in the context of national policy; secondly,

> at the level where the national policies are applied to local circumstances – for example, between Regional Boards and Boards of Governors, to ensure an integrated hospital service in both teaching and non-teaching hospitals; between Regional Boards, Boards of Governors and local health authorities to secure an efficiently planned and organised maternity service; between hospital authorities, local authorities (both health and welfare) and Executive Councils to plan an integrated service for the care and treatment of the aged, etc.

and, thirdly, at the personal level between individual health workers.[5]

Accepting for a moment the Guillebaud Committee's analysis, the responsibility of the Leeds Board lay at the second level. However, the Board's attempts to facilitate co-ordination did not always meet with success. This was certainly true of the Regional Liaison Committee, which after an active beginning gradually came to meet less frequently. In 1956 the Board's Chairman drew attention to this, commenting that the requirement that the Committee meet at six-monthly intervals 'was more frequent than the present volume of business warranted'. He pointed out that the last occasion a constituent authority other than the Board had submitted an item for the agenda was October 1954. While he hoped that this would change, thus enabling the Committee to meet at least once every six months, he proposed that the constitution should be amended to require only annual meetings, and this was agreed. Thereafter the Committee met at approximately twelve-monthly intervals but, in view of the continued shortage of agenda items and the low attendance rate, it was questionable whether even meetings of this frequency were justified. One of the consequences of the Committee's decline was that the Medical Officers of Health Liaison Committee again became the main link between the Board and local authorities. For the most part, however, the Committee was concerned with what were essentially medical matters, like the arrangements to be made in the event of a smallpox epidemic, rather than wider health and welfare issues, such as the health needs of the mentally ill.

In contrast to the regional position, there were a number of encouraging local developments, and it is here that it is possible to take the Guillebaud Committee's analysis further. Tibbitt has suggested that liaison between agencies in the health and welfare field can be analysed at three levels: co-operation between professionals over individual cases; operational co-ordination over particular services; and strategic planning.[6] Operational co-ordination and strategic planning can be seen as sub-divisions of the Guillebaud Committee's second category of liaison, the application of national policy to local circumstances, and, in terms of the formal division of functions in the NHS, it might be expected that joint strategic planning would fall within the ambit of regional boards and local health authorities, and operational co-ordination would be undertaken by hospital management committees and local health authorities.

What we have argued so far is that contacts between the Board and local health authorities were uneven in both frequency and direction. As far as content was concerned, a number of issues were discussed, including the interchange of staff and the development of child guidance services. But what of the quality of discussions? Towell has postulated a range of different approaches to planning by two or more agencies: unconnected planning, independent planning based on shared information, joint bargaining and joint planning.[7] In the Leeds Region the predominant mode was unconnected planning by the Board and local health authorities, with in a few instances information being exchanged, and, exceptionally, joint bargaining taking place, for example over the arrangements to be made in the child guidance service, where local authorities agreed to provide the premises, psychologists and social workers at child guidance clinics, and the Board made available the services of consultant psychiatrists.

Operational co-ordination between hospital management committees and local health authorities followed a similar pattern, although there were a number of more positive developments. In the maternity service, for example, local maternity liaison committees were set up throughout the Region in accordance with the recommendations of the Cranbrook Committee, which reported in 1959.[8] Again, in mental health the hospital and local authority services worked closely together in Hull, Leeds and York. In Hull a jointly staffed and funded day centre was provided; in Leeds the acute psychiatric unit developed at St James's Hospital during the 1950s housed local authority mental health workers as well as hospital staff;

and, in York, a comprehensive mental health service which attracted wide attention was provided by the local authority and the hospital management committee.[9] Also, as we have already mentioned, there was good operational co-ordination in Leeds over geriatric services. Co-operation between professionals in respect of individual cases was a feature of a number of these initiatives, with case conferences complementing the more formal joint committee arrangements at the operational level.

The Health and Welfare Plan and after

As the NHS moved into its second decade, the importance of liaison was once more underlined by the passing of the Mental Health Act in 1959, and by the development of long-term plans for the hospital service and local authority services. With its emphasis on care in the community, the 1959 Act placed a much greater responsibility on local authorities to make provision for the mentally ill. In particular, the permissive powers available to authorities under Section 28 of the National Health Service Act of 1946 were made mandatory, and consequently a considerable expansion of local authority homes and hostels was envisaged. At the same time, effective joint action by hospital authorities and local authorities was seen as being crucial to the success of the new policy. However, a survey of the local response to the Act carried out by the Board in 1960 indicated some of the barriers to liaison. For example, one of the proposals made by the Ministry of Health was that there should be joint appointments of psychiatric social workers and mental health welfare workers. These appointments were not thought desirable by HMCs and local authorities. Again, the modesty of local authorities' revised proposals for services to be provided under Section 28 of the NHS Act created doubts as to whether the shift from hospital to community care could become a reality.

These doubts were reinforced by the white paper, *Health and Welfare: The Development of Community Care*, published in April 1963.[10] The white paper was the local authorities' counterpart of the Hospital Plan, and it contained summaries of the services which each local health and welfare authority was planning to provide in 1967 and 1972. Although these summaries were preceded by a commentary by the Ministry, the Health and Welfare Plan has rightly been described as 'a collation of the relatively independent predictions, intentions or ambitions of departments in 146 individual authorities'.[11] As the Ministry of Health explained, the reason for this was that: 'Each authority has an independent responsibility in its own area, and no attempt was made to indicate common standards to which the plans should conform or to suggest modifications before publication'.[12]

In the absence of common standards, there were wide variations in the proposed provision of staff and accommodation, and Table 7.1 indicates some of the variations among authorities in the Leeds Region. To take two specific examples: the places in homes for the elderly per thousand of population aged 65 and over proposed for 1972 ranged from 14.5 in the East Riding to 42.3 in Leeds, and the number of health visitors per thousand of population proposed for 1972 ranged from 0.09 in the East Riding and the West Riding to 0.23 in Bradford. Neither the uneven development of complementary hospital and voluntary services nor the different needs of local populations could satisfactorily explain such wide variations.

The Leeds Board, in considering the plans prior to publication, was concerned that these variations would hinder implementation of the Hospital Plan. The Board gave as an example services for the elderly, pointing out that the reduction in geriatric bed provision in the Region from 1.7 beds per thousand population to the norm of 1.3 beds per thousand set in the Hospital Plan was unlikely to be achieved because some local authorities were not proposing to build up places in old people's homes at a fast enough rate. The Board therefore asked the Ministry to establish targets of provision for local authorities, and this was done in the Health and Welfare Plan. For example, as far as residential accommodation for the elderly was concerned, a target of between 18 and 22 places per thousand population aged 65 and over was set.

One of the express intentions of the Plan was, in fact, 'to stimulate discussion, study and experiment, and make it possible for local authorities to consider and revise their own intentions in the light of what others are doing and proposing'.[13] Hence, revisions of plans were likely to be more significant than the original plans, as comparison would lead to amendments, and, it was hoped, greater uniformity. The extent to which this happened is shown in Table 7.2, which indicates some of the variations among authorities in the Leeds Region, drawn from the revised Health and Welfare Plan published in June 1966.

TABLE 7.1 *Variations in the standard of provision planned by local authorities in the Leeds Region*

	Places in training centres for mentally subnormal/ 1000 pop. planned for 1972		Places in homes for the elderly 1000 pop. over 65 planned for 1972	Health visitors/ 1000 pop. planned for 1972	Home helps/ 1000 pop. planned for 1972	Home nurses/ 1000 pop. planned for 1972	Midwives/ 1000 pop. planned for 1972	Social workers/ 1000 pop. planned for 1972
	Junior	Adult						
National average	0.46	0.55	20.0	0.15	0.73	0.19	0.13	0.10
Regional average	0.55	0.63	28.87	0.18	0.90	0.24	0.11	0.14
Range within region	0.20 →0.95	0.40 →1.11	14.5–42.3	0.09–0.23	0.48–1.31	0.16–0.47	0.04–0.20	0.06–0.23

SOURCE *Health and Welfare: The Development of Community Care*, Cmnd. 1973 (London: HMSO, 1963). Compiled from the tables on pp. 79–99 and pp. 366–7.

TABLE 7.2 *Variations in the standard of provision planned by local authorities in the Leeds Region*

	Places in training centres for mentally subnormal/1000 pop. planned for 1972		Places in homes for the elderly/1000 pop. over 65 planned for 1972	Health visitors/1000 pop. planned for 1972	Home helps/1000 pop. planned for 1972	Home nurses/1000 pop. planned for 1972	Midwives/1000 pop. planned for 1972	Social workers/1000 pop. planned for 1972
	Junior	Adult						
National average	0.54	0.65	21.7	0.17	0.85	0.20	0.13	0.12
Regional average	0.61	0.65	26.03	0.18	1.12	0.23	0.11	0.13
Range within region	0.40 ↓ 0.94	0.29 ↓ 0.96	16.0–32.2	0.12–0.24	0.71–1.59	0.15–0.50	0.05–0.19	0.05–0.19

SOURCE *Health and Welfare: The Development of Community Care*, Cmnd. 3022 (London: HMSO, 1966). Compiled from tables on pp. 59–79 and pp. 412–13.

While the variations were, on the whole, smaller than in 1963, large differences still remained, and it is clear that the movement towards uniformity was occurring only slowly. Significantly, in the revised Plan the Ministry announced its intention to take a tougher line with backward authorities. It stated:

> Where the provision of a service appears to be substantially below an adequate level and likely to remain so over the whole period of the present plans, the Minister proposes to arrange for his officers to discuss the position with the authority concerned with a view to action to remedy any deficiency.[14]

Despite this statement, there is no convincing evidence that the Ministry did in fact adopt a more interventionist stance. Griffith, for instance, has described the Ministry's attitude to local health and welfare authorities as 'laissez-faire', which he defines as 'as little interference as is possible within the necessary fulfillment of departmental duties'.[15] And Judge has shown how local autonomy rather than territorial justice has been the dominant value in the administration of local health and welfare services.[16] This shows an interesting contrast between the Ministry's relationship with local health authorities on the one hand and hospital authorities on the other – a theme developed further in Chapter 8.

Notwithstanding variations in standards, preparation of the plans has been called 'an event of great significance for the future development of the service'.[17] Following Brown,[18] it can be said that the Ministry's request to local authorities to submit development programmes had several effects: it encouraged a systematic rather than an incremental approach to the development of services; it drew attention to norms which, while not mandatory, were presented as desirable targets; it provided officers with a basis on which to draw up plans for their committee; within each authority it strengthened the claim of health and welfare services for a greater share of resources; and publication of the plans provided a means of comparing the intentions of authorities and highlighting those with low aspirations.

Another effect noticeable in the Leeds Region was to give the Regional Liaison Committee something to talk about. This is not to suggest that the Committee influenced what went into local authorities' plans. Far from it; for the extent of the Committee's and the Board's involvement was to be informed of local authorities' proposals in advance. Independent planning based on shared information describes this process well. Yet the Liaison Committee continued to struggle to find a role, and to meet only annually. In 1964 the Board suggested that less frequent meetings should be considered in view of the existence of a number of other forms of liaison, such as the Medical Officers of Health Liaison Committee. The minutes record that 'members felt that the meetings provided for a very useful exchange of information between the Board and Local Authorities and that the Committee should continue to meet annually'. Ironically, this proved to be the final entry in the Committee's minutes, for in the event no further meetings were held.

After 1964 what contact there was with local authorities occurred either through bilateral meetings, or through the medical officers of health. Yet the value of the latter channel of liaison was considerably lessened in 1971, when the Local Authority Social Services Act of 1970 came into operation. The Act, which was based on the recommendations of the Seebohm Committee,[19] brought together under a single local authority committee and department the services previously administered by the welfare and children's departments, and some of the services of the health departments. Decisions on which local authority health services should be transferred to the new departments were based on the principle that services primarily involving social work skills should be transferred, while those involving mainly medical skills should be retained. The newly unified personal social services were in this way separated from community health services like health centres, health education and vaccination and immunisation. Another important consequence of the Seebohm reforms was that social workers, instead of specialising in work with particular clients like children or the mentally ill as they had done in the past, were henceforth expected to provide a family service by taking on a 'generic' caseload.

These reforms are usually seen as a victory for the emerging social work profession over the medical officers of health, many of whose functions, including services for the mentally disordered, were transferred to the new Directors of Social Services. Certainly, local government medical officers put up a spirited resistance to the social work lobby, though Hall has warned that 'it would be wrong to see the clash of interests over Seebohm as involving a straight fight between the medical profession and social workers'.[20] Nevertheless, the medical officers' reservations about the separation of social and medical care were shared by many health service personnel, particularly consultant psychiatrists. Experience after 1971 showed some of these fears to be justified. For example, a report to the Board in 1972 indicated that psychiatrists were facing difficulties because generic social workers often lacked psychiatric experience; there had been a reduction in the number of social workers engaged full-time in mental health; and there were consequent problems in finding suitably qualified social workers to deal with emergencies. To some extent these problems could be explained in terms of the teething troubles of a new service; an alternative view was that the reforms were ill-conceived and created more difficulties than they solved. At the least there seemed to be a good case for delaying the reforms for three years until the simultaneous reorganisation of local government and the NHS. Whatever the interpretation, what is not in question is that the Seebohm reorganisation created immediate difficulties for the hospital service at the level of inter-professional co-operation.

Likewise, there is no evidence that the reorganisation led to more effective liaison in the strategic planning of services. This can be seen from the response to the 1971 white paper, *Better Services for the Mentally Handicapped*,[21] which asked hospital authorities and local authorities to plan jointly their mental handicap services. As Jones and her colleagues comment in their study of these services in the Region:

> In 1972 and 1973 the Regional Hospital Board took the initiative in approaching Directors of Social Services, drawing their attention to the White Paper proposals and calling meetings for discussion; but the response so far has been less than enthusiastic.[22]

Liaison was again limited to independent planning based on shared information, and this applied to all services, not just those for the mentally handicapped.

Liaison with executive councils

As in the case of local authorities, liaison between the Board and executive councils was effected in a number of ways. First, there was overlapping membership. Secondly, a medical advisory committee on the General Practitioner/Hospital Service relationship was set up in 1952. The committee comprised a nominee from each local medical committee and other practitioners nominated by the Board. It functioned alongside other medical advisory committees as an advisory body to the officers, the Specialist Services Advisory Committee, and ultimately the Board. A third channel of liaison was opened up in 1953, when executive councils were invited to send six representatives to the Regional Liaison Committee of the Board and local authorities. At the same time the Board of Governors of the United Leeds Hospitals was also invited to nominate representatives, and so the Committee became a forum for all health service authorities in the Region. Finally, liaison was promoted less formally by the SAMO and his assistants, who regularly attended meetings of local medical committees.

The main issue involving the Board and GPs in the early years of the NHS was the future of cottage hospitals. Before 1948 almost all work in cottage hospitals was done by GPs with the occasional assistance of visiting specialists. The advent of the NHS, with its promise of freely available specialist skills, raised the question of whether these arrangements should continue. A report to the Board in September 1949 addressed this question and detailed two options: cottage hospitals could be regarded as an essential part of the hospital service and an important link between general practitioners and hospitals, in which case they should be provided in urban as well as rural areas; or they could be regarded as a special provision to meet the needs of small population groups in rural areas. The report noted that the Board had tended to follow the latter policy and recommended that it should continue to do so. This was accepted. Minimum criteria for defining a cottage hospital were then laid down: it should have no resident medical staff and not more than 50 beds; it should be situated at least 10 miles from a general hospital; and it should cater for all the commoner, less serious types of illness. Adopting these criteria, the Board decided that nine cottage hospitals should continue to function as such; four with larger bed complements should be upgraded to small general hospitals with resident staff; and six near to general hospitals should be affiliated to these hospitals and become annexes to them. A considerable reduction in general practitioner work in hospitals was therefore planned.

However, two weeks after taking these decisions the Board received a circular setting out the Ministry's views on the role of cottage hospitals.[23] The circular stressed the need for full consultation with general practitioners and the public when Boards were contemplating a change in status, and asked hospital authorities:

> to make sure that in carrying out their plans they are not depriving local patients of a valuable feature of the general practitioner (cottage) hospital; i.e. its use as a local hospital to which the general practitioners of the neighbourhood can admit patients who require treatment within the scope of a general practitioner but who, for various good reasons, cannot be treated at home.

The circular reminded Boards of the Minister's reserve powers 'to call upon a Board to report to him their reasons for adopting their new policy'.

The Leeds Board, acting before this advice was issued, had not proceeded as recommended. In particular, it had failed to consult local interests and was proposing a reduction in the number of cottage hospitals in the Region. When its plans became known they drew strong protests from several areas. Conflict centred on the Lloyd Hospital, Bridlington, the Skipton General Hospital, and the Bingley and District Hospital, which the Board proposed to upgrade to small general hospitals; and on the Holme Valley Memorial Hospital, Huddersfield, and the Sir Titus Salt's Hospital, Shipley, which the Board wanted to affiliate to established general hospitals. The Ministry intervened and requested the Board to defer implementation of its policy until objections had been heard. The Ministry also asked to be kept informed of developments so that it could comment on any final decision before it was made public.

Following detailed investigations into the circumstances surrounding each hospital, and after ascertaining the views of local general practitioners and members of HMCs, the Board produced revised proposals. In the case of the Holme Valley Memorial Hospital and the Sir Titus Salt's Hospital it decided to abandon affiliation and to allow the hospitals to continue as cottage hospitals. The position at the remaining three hospitals was more complicated, but eventually an agreement was reached with the general practitioners at the Lloyd Hospital and this was then applied to the other two. The basis of the agreement was that the hospitals would become small general hospitals, but the general practitioners would be appointed as clinical assistants and would perform the duties required of hospital medical officers and house officers as well as the duties usually associated with clinical assistants. They would be allowed to give anaesthetics to their own patients and assist as far as practicable at operations, but agreed to acknowledge that ultimate clinical responsibility rested with consultants. The acceptability of these arrangements was due in no small part to the fact that the GPs concerned were to be paid not only at the clinical assistant rate but also out of a special fund set up for each hospital. This system of remuneration gave considerable financial benefits to the GPs.

Once the future of cottage hospitals had been decided, very few issues of concern to executive councils and GPs came on to the Board's agenda. A number of commentators have remarked on the widening gulf between primary care and hospital care with the advent of the NHS,[24] and our data do not contradict this judgement. Separation was not of course complete, and GPs continued to be employed in hospitals as clinical assistants. As well as furthering links between the hospital and general practitioner services, clinical assistants made an important contribution to medical staffing in hospitals. This contribution was especially significant in regions like Leeds which often found it difficult to recruit junior doctors. In 1962 the Board employed the whole-time equivalent of 63 GPs, more than any other region except Birmingham.[25] This figure had doubled by 1973, and the increase was in large part accounted for by the restrictions imposed in 1967 on the expansion of the registrar grade. Clinical assistants were in many cases substitutes for registrars, and as such made a significant contribution to the staffing of the hospital service.[26]

Hospital appointments apart, GPs were also concerned to have access to diagnostic facilities, and to maternity beds. As early as 1952 the Board informed local medical committees of its policy of allowing GPs the use of pathological and radiological facilities 'wherever accommodation could be made available', adding that 'facilities would be extended as soon as accommodation was available at the hospitals where the facilities did not exist'. An indication of the increasing use and availability of these facilities is that the number of direct referrals to x-ray departments rose from 78 000 in 1955 to 194 000 in 1971.

On maternity beds, the Board followed the Ministry of Health's recommendation that GPs should be permitted access in the smaller but not the larger maternity units. This meant that GPs in rural areas were most favoured, and a 1952 survey indicated that none of the maternity beds in the Airedale, Wharfedale and East Riding areas was closed to GPs. The same survey found that 28 per cent of the maternity beds in the Region was open to GPs, and between 1954 and 1973 the number of designated GP maternity beds increased from 118 to 326.

In pursuing these policies the Board was very much in line with the recommendations of the Cohen Report,[27] published in 1954, and the Gillie Report,[28] published in 1963. The Gillie Report was the general practitioners' counterpart to the Hospital Plan and the Health and Welfare Plan, in that it looked at the future work of the family doctor having regard to the development of hospital and local authority services. The longest chapter in the Report concerned 'the interdependence of the family doctor and the hospital service', and it advocated hospital appointments for GPs and direct access to diagnostic services. Also emphasised was the need for GPs to be allocated hospital beds, and the Report noted that this facility had not previously been available to most family doctors in urban areas. Accordingly, it recommended that: 'Boards should be encouraged to experiment in the use of general practitioner beds at existing acute general hospitals before the new district hospitals envisaged in the Hospital Plan are built.'[29]

The Leeds Board responded by setting up a special working party which reported in October 1965. The working party's main proposal was that a pilot scheme should be launched in which a definite allocation of acute beds in a general hospital would be made to family doctors. The aim of the scheme would be to assess the use made of the beds and the type of work done in order that the need for GP beds in the planned network of district general hospitals could be more closely defined. The Board gave its approval to the scheme, which was eventually started in 1968 at Staincliffe General Hospital, Dewsbury. Medical beds at the Hospital were made available to GPs working under the overall control of the consultant physician.

However, in the first year of operation only two patients were treated by their own GPs. Subsequent years brought little improvement, despite repeated attempts to publicise the availability of the beds. Although the scheme was not evaluated, those to whom we spoke felt that its failure could be attributed to the heavy workload of GPs in the Dewsbury area; the reluctance of junior hospital doctors to provide the necessary cover; and the fact that the GPs received no payment for the work. These factors, which bore out the Gillie Report's observation that any such scheme was likely to meet 'administrative, clinical and personality difficulties',[30] militated against the experiment being an effective link between general and specialist practice.

Much more encouraging in this respect was the increasing involvement of hospitals in the vocational training of GPs. During the 1960s it came to be recognised that the traditional form of entry into general practice – successful completion of the undergraduate medical course followed by a year's hospital experience – was no longer adequate preparation for a complex field of work. Thus both the Royal College of General Practitioners and the Royal Commission on Medical Education, which reported in 1968,[31] advocated more rigorous and extensive professional training. Consequently, in the Leeds Region an advisory committee on general practice to the Standing Joint Committee on Postgraduate Medical Education was set up in 1970, and part-time tutors in general practice were appointed in each of the four postgraduate areas. Two years later vocational training schemes were in operation in York and Airedale, and others were planned for Leeds, Wakefield, Hull, Harrogate and Pontefract. Training typically extended over three years, during which time four periods of rotating hospital appointments in senior house officer posts were sandwiched between two periods of general practice appointments. While most of the trainees' time in hospitals was spent in established posts and so did not require additional funding, the Board made money available to cover the cost of gaps between the starting dates of service posts, and in addition a number of special, non-established posts were created. As well as representing a significant investment in the future of general practice, the development of these schemes helped to build early and potentially lasting bridges between family doctors and their hospital colleagues.

Conclusion

In conclusion, the first point to note about liaison between the Board and local health authorities is that those involved were mainly officers rather than members. Among officers, it was the medical officers on both sides who were the principal participants, with liaison primarily being conducted in the interstices of the Board's medical advisory committee system. Members did play a part, both on the Board itself and on the Regional Liaison Committee, but the latter was a dismal failure. What lay behind this failure, and does the Committee's impotence hold more general lessons for inter-organisational relationships in the NHS?

It will be recalled that the Committee was set up in 1951 after the West Riding County Council had objected to the Board's obtaining advice from local authorities primarily through medical officers of health. The Committee was thus seen as a safeguard against possible officer domination of joint discussions. But it was also an experiment in liaison, for at the time of its formation the newly established hospital authorities were viewed with some suspicion by local authorities, and there was little evidence to show how the two types of authority might best co-ordinate their activities in a Service still very much in its infancy. It was therefore implicit in the Committee's origins that, if officer domination did not result, and if other means of collaboration were found to be more effective, then the Committee would no longer be needed.

The decision to enlarge the Committee's membership to include representatives of executive councils and the Board of Governors of the United Leeds Hospitals resulted in a large body expected to cover all aspects of collaboration. Again, the Committee was purely advisory, any recommendations having to be approved by constituent authorities. It was not an appropriate forum for reaching agreement on issues which required immediate action. It gradually became apparent, then, that liaison was not best achieved by a Committee of all four types of health authority organised at regional level, with the remit of discussing any matters of common interest, and without executive powers. What happened was that the Committee came to meet less frequently, agenda items all came from the Board, and at best meetings enabled an exchange of information to take place. In practice there was no joint strategic planning of services, and there appeared to be no incentives for such planning to develop.

. Far more effective were the experiments in operational co-ordination launched in various parts of the Region, like the liaison committee for mental health services in York and for geriatric services in Leeds. These succeeded where the Regional Liaison Committee failed because they were concerned with more practical issues of day-to-day co-ordination; they were area- rather than region-based; and they were involved with a particular service. Also, as Jones has noted, successful examples of liaison tended to occur where the areas of hospital and local authority boundaries were broadly the same, and where there was a political and professional commitment to joint working.[32] The last point was especially important, with the stimulus provided by a medical officer of health or a consultant often being the crucial factor. As we have remarked, it was in those areas where operational co-ordination was most advanced that inter-professional collaboration over individual cases was also well developed.

The Leeds and York experiments were, however, exceptional rather than typical, and locally as well as regionally the dominant approach to liaison, in terms of Towell's typology, was at best shared information, rather than real joint planning and co-ordination of services. It does not therefore make sense to ask how joint policies were made and implemented, whose will prevailed in joint discussions, how problems were defined, and so on, because the relationship was not of this kind. There were occasions when the Board engaged in bargaining with local authorities – for example, over child guidance services – and the outcome of these situations was usually a compromise between the wishes of the Board and the authority concerned. Otherwise the planning of hospital and local health authority services tended to occur along parallel lines.

Like the dog who did not bark in the night, this is something to be explained. Part of the answer, as already indicated, is that there was no apparent incentive to undertake joint activity. Having assessed the likely outcome of joint planning and operational co-ordination in relation to the investment of time required, it can be argued that the Board, HMCs and local health authorities decided that participation was not worthwhile. In other words, if relationships between organisations are seen in terms of exchange, then hospital and local health authorities concluded that they had more to lose than to gain from joint planning. However plausible this explanation may be, it falls too easily into the language and assumptions of the rational actor model.[33] The absence of joint activity may indeed have been the result of rational calculation, but before this is put forward as the decisive reason alternative explanations need to be considered. One alternative would emphasise the importance of organisational factors, arguing that the mismatch between the Board and HMCs on the one hand, and local health authorities on the other, in terms of their membership, officer structure, committee systems, financing and so on, seemed designed to frustrate joint planning and operational co-ordination. Another alternative would attribute failures in liaison to political factors. For example, the Regional Liaison Committee was advisory and not executive, it lacked political 'clout', and it therefore attracted little interest from senior members of the Board and local authorities. Only when there was a political commitment did joint activity really work. Each of these models – the rational, organisational and political – helps explain why liaison developed as it did.

As we hope to have demonstrated, relationships between the Board and GPs did not figure prominently on the Board's agenda, apart from the early attempt to rationalise cottage hospitals. Like a number of the Board's other initial ventures in the planning field, this was an attempt to find a rational solution to some of the problems of the hospital service, and it failed for the same reason: opposition from local professionals. The eventual outcome was the result of adjustment between the wishes of these professionals and the Board's officers. This issue aside, liaison was managed at a low-key level by the medical advisory committee on the general practitioner hospital service relationship. The committee was again a forum for the exchange and sharing of information, rather than a mechanism for taking major policy decisions. As the Board explained in its *Review of Policy and Objectives* published in 1968, while the committee:

> has been of great value in keeping the general practitioners appraised of Board policy and for discussing matters of detailed difficulty arising in local medical committees it does not . . . consider any of the fundamental issues affecting the future relationships with the hospital service.

Given the independent position occupied by GPs in the NHS, it was not perhaps surprising that it was in this area of liaison that joint activity was least in evidence.

8

Centre–periphery Relationships

In all public services in which administrative responsibility is shared between a central authority and locally based authorities there is a need to strike a balance between the powers and functions of the centre and those of the periphery. The purpose of this chapter is to examine the nature of the balance that was struck between the Ministry of Health (and later DHSS) and regional hospital boards. The chapter proceeds from a general overview of central department/regional board relationships, through an examination of the means of central control, making use of material from the Leeds Region, to an analysis of the relationship which draws on the literature on central government/local government relations.

It should be noted that, while the centre has been defined as the Ministry of Health and DHSS, it is important to take account of the influence of other central agencies, in particular the Treasury, and this is done at a number of points in the chapter. Also, the periphery comprised not just RHBs but also the boards of governors of teaching hospitals, and hospital management committees. Boards of governors were in an unusual position in that they normally covered a similar area to HMCs, but combined the functions of HMCs and RHBs and were in direct contact with the central department. Their role is not considered, however, because no data are available.

On the other hand, there is some discussion of HMCs, and their place in the structure of administrative control. But the main emphasis throughout the chapter is on the relationship between the central department and regional boards, with evidence from the Leeds Region being used to illustrate and amplify the general argument which is based mainly on official reports and other published material.

Overview

Guidance on the kind of relationship envisaged by the Ministry of Health came in the first NHS circular, RHB(47)1, which referred to regional boards as the Minister's agents, adding that the Minister wanted boards 'to feel from the outset . . . a lively sense of independent responsibility'. HMCs were described as the boards' agents, and the circular stressed that

> the Minister wants these Committees to enjoy the maximum of autonomy in regard to local day-to-day administration, reserving power to the Boards to decide questions of wider policy, to control major building operations, to approve the Committee's budgets and other similar functions.

Later circulars, such as HM(69)59 issued after the Ely Report, did little more than reiterate the agency principle, which remained ill-defined.

However, DHSS was more forthcoming in evidence to the Expenditure Committee of the House of Commons. There it was stated that the role of DHSS was to control total expenditure, issue guidance on broad policy and priorities and approve certain key expenditure decisions. Consequently, the Department 'seeks to avoid interfering in decisions proper to regional or local hospital management'.[1] An interesting parallel was drawn between the administration of the hospital service and the local authority social services. Local authorities were seen as 'independent of the Department',[2] the major instrument of central control being the rate support grant. In contrast, 'the influence of the Department means something more direct in the case of the National Health Service, certainly the hospital side of it, than it does in the case of local authorities'.[3]

These statements suggest a relationship of central control mediated by regional and local autonomy. Certain factors, like the accountability to Parliament of the Minister of Health (later the Secretary of State for Social Services), the absence of any local sources of revenue, and the central appointment of board members, favoured central control. Other factors, like the system of block rather than earmarked grants, the appointment to boards and committees of local 'notables', and the superior local knowledge of board and committee members and officers, worked in the opposite direction. A sort of system of checks and balances was in operation, with the scales not weighed heavily either to the centre or the periphery.

It is interesting to compare this interpretation with the views of Enoch Powell, Minister of Health between 1960 and 1963, and Richard Crossman, Secretary of State for Social Services between 1968 and 1970. It was Powell's view that boards were 'an administrative chain for the transmission of central policy and decision', and that 'the interposition of the regional hospital boards between the hospital management committees and the Minister has even paradoxically had the effect of rendering centralisation more rigid'.[4] In direct contrast, Richard Crossman described the relationship between his Department and boards thus:

> You have a number of powerful, semi-autonomous Boards whose relation to me was much more like the relations of a Persian satrap to a weak Persian Emperor. If the Emperor tried to enforce his authority too far he lost his throne or at least he lost his resources or something broke down. In much the same way Health Service freedom lies in the fact that the centre is weak and the Regional Hospital Boards are strong.[5]

Significantly, the second green paper on NHS reorganisation, published when Crossman was Secretary of State, stated that in the reorganised Service 'the central Department will need to concern itself more closely than in the past with the expenditure and the efficiency of the administration at the local level'.[6]

Here then are three different interpretations of central department/regional board relationships: Powell's emphasises central control; Crossman's stresses regional autonomy; and the official view suggests a relationship somewhere in between. To shed light on which interpretation is the most plausible, consideration will be given to the development of the relationship between 1948 and 1974, and to the various means by which control was or was not exercised over specific areas of service provision.

The relationship over time

In the years immediately after 1948 tight controls were imposed on boards. The main reason for this was financial, and it is here that Treasury influence was most evident. In 1948 and again in 1949 NHS expenditure exceeded estimates, and in the following year an expenditure ceiling was introduced. At the same time, the Ministry of Health introduced restrictions on hospital staffing and finance. Boards were required to obtain the Ministry's approval before appointing new staff, and one result was that control over additional consultant posts was transferred to the centre. On finance, monthly returns of expenditure had to be sent to the Ministry and boards were deprived of the power to approve transfers between the subheadings of management committees' expenditure. In addition, the Ministry's principal regional officers began attending board meetings as observers and receiving minutes and papers.

Commenting on these controls, the House of Commons Estimates Committee, in a report published in 1951, advised that the Ministry should decide whether to allow boards greater autonomy or to make them primarily planning and advisory bodies, as they were tending to become.[7] In the event the former option was chosen, and from the early 1950s onwards central controls were gradually relaxed. As the Guillebaud Committee noted in 1956, 'since 1951 . . . there has been a gradual building up of the Regional Hospital Boards both in the financial and other fields'.[8] An example of this was that boards were given global financial allocations and the power of virement was restored to them. However, Guillebaud argued that still more could be done to enhance the authority of boards: 'We are of the opinion that the primary need now is to give more emphasis . . . to the Regional Board's responsibility for the general oversight and supervision of the service (in addition to their planning functions)'.[9] This advice was followed, and in 1959, for example, the remaining controls over non-medical hospital staff were removed.

In the 1960s the Ministry and boards moved forward together. This partnership was most evident in relation to the Hospital Plan of 1962. The initiative taken by the Ministry in asking boards to prepare ten-year development plans was universally welcomed as an example of the creative leadership which many observers felt was lacking in the hospital service in the 1950s.[10] Of particular importance was the success of the Permanent Secretary, Sir Bruce Fraser, in persuading the Treasury to sanction a plan estimated to cost £500 million over 10 years. In responding positively to the Ministry's initiative boards came into their own as planning bodies for the first time. The extension of boards' supervisory powers in the 1950s was therefore complemented by an extension of their planning responsibilities in the 1960s.

The Hospital Plan was very much a joint effort. The Ministry issued guidance detailing the concept of the district general hospital and the bed norms to be used in planning new hospitals. In addition advice on design was issued in the form of Building Notes, and these Notes were essentially 'a distillation of current and best practice'[11] of boards. Officers of the department collaborated with boards' officers in planning particular projects, and major schemes required departmental approval. Subject to these controls, and within the budgets allocated to them, boards were left free to choose where and when to undertake new building. In this way a balance was struck between central control and local autonomy.

In the late 1960s this balance was upset by the series of enquiries into conditions at long-stay hospitals which began with Ely.[12] Following the Ely report the Department asked boards to consider diverting capital and revenue funds to long-stay services. When boards replied that this was impossible within existing allocations, the Department followed the example set in the development of renal dialysis units by earmarking money specifically for these services. At the same time guidance was issued on minimum standards to be achieved at long-stay hospitals, and the Hospital Advisory Service was established to visit and report on those hospitals. The Service was described as the Secretary of State's 'eyes and ears' and it reported directly to him. By these means the Department, having discovered the limits of its control, attempted to enhance that control.

Thus, to summarise this brief overview of board/department relations between 1948 and 1974, the early years were characterised by central control; during the 1950s this control was relaxed and boards were given greater freedom; in the 1960s the department and boards moved forward together; and in the years immediately before reorganisation there was a movement back towards centralisation.

The means of control

The discussion can be taken a stage further by examining the means by which central control was exercised. These were of various kinds. On finance, for example, the department had complete control over the total budget of the hospital service and the allocation of the budget between boards, subject of course to Treasury and Cabinet decisions on the size and distribution of public expenditure as a whole. This qualification is important because the rate of growth of government spending and decisions on priorities between programme areas clearly had an impact on the hospital service. Nowhere is this better illustrated than by the hospital building programme, which did not take off until 1962 because up to that date greater priority was given to other areas of capital investment – like housing, education and defence. Only when there was a central government commitment to hospital building did this change.

It was, however, left to the Ministry of Health and DHSS to decide how to distribute the total budget between boards, and throughout the period 1948–74 there continued to be wide variations in *per capita* expenditure between regions. These variations are evidence not of regional autonomy but of the centre's lack of concern to promote territorial justice. As the former Minister of State for Health, David Owen, has written: 'The department's central responsibility for redressing inequalities has been woefully neglected'.[13] This is one of the more significant ways in which the NHS differs from local government, where disparities in the level of service provision do indicate local autonomy.[14]

In contrast with the department's control over the allocation of expenditure between regions, there was no central control over the distribution of this expenditure within regions, which was a matter for boards alone to decide. Of course, boards were guided in their decisions by the policy advice issued by the department, but the effect of this advice was limited by historical factors. The bulk of revenue expenditure allocated by boards each year was inherited expenditure. If the department asked boards to give priority to long-stay services, as it did in the late 1960s, then this could only be achieved by additional funding. As we explained in Chapter 5, in 1969 HMCs in the Leeds Region made it clear that they were opposed to any diversion of revenue from general hospitals to long-stay hospitals within existing budgets, and this message was passed on by the Leeds Board to the DHSS.

It was for this reason that extra, earmarked sums were set aside for long-stay services starting in 1970. Similar considerations applied to capital expenditure, with most of the capital programme each year being taken up with schemes already under way. It inevitably took time for departmental advice to work its way through into the capital programme. As one of the department's officers conceded in evidence to the Estimates Committee: 'Although we might be pushing a Board in one direction, the extent to which we can push it in any one year is limited by this budgeting arrangement'.[15] On both capital and revenue, then, the department's overall control was mediated by boards' decisions on the distribution of funds made available to them. The only precise means of control open to the department was earmarking, and this was used sparingly. In any case, later experience of earmarking money for the building of regional secure units for the mentally ill demonstrated that this method was only an incentive and could not guarantee the implementation of national policy goals.

A clearer move towards centralisation is apparent in relation to medical manpower. At the inception of the NHS all medical appointments were made either by boards or management committees. From 1952 onwards approval was required for appointments in the consultant, senior hospital medical officer and senior registrar grades, and this was later extended to the registrar grade. The establishment in 1972 of the Central Manpower Committee was a further move in the same direction, and the Committee now theoretically controls the distribution and growth of almost all hospital doctor grades.[16]

A general instrument of departmental control was the use of circulars giving guidance and advice on service developments. In this context, 'control' may be too strong a word for two reasons. First, most circulars did not simply descend from above but were the outcome of prior consultation between boards and the department. This is indicated by the Leeds Board's objection to circular RHB(50)80 on the ground that 'the issue of an important directive without prior consultation with regional hospital boards is a procedure which is contrary to well established practice'. Secondly, the impact made by circulars was questionable, as Brown showed in 1962.[17] Brown traced the course of a circular on hospital catering in 16 HMCs and found that, although reactions varied, in general little attention was given to the circular and few of its recommendations were adopted. Eight months after Brown's survey the Ministry announced the introduction of pink-coloured circulars. The main features of these circulars were that copies were to be given to members of boards; board secretaries were to ensure that relevant staff received copies and not only took action on the circulars but also reported that action; and the Ministry was to be informed of the action taken. A form of monitoring was therefore introduced in an attempt to make circulars serve their purpose more effectively. Yet, as Stewart and Sleeman showed in a study of the response to a pink circular on out-patient departments, issued in 1964, there was little evidence that pink circulars were more effective.[18] Hence, as a means of increased central control this instrument was of doubtful utility.

One of the functions served by circulars was to give guidance on different standards of provision which the central department wanted boards and management committees to follow. The most common of these standards were bed norms specifying the number of beds to be provided in a given specialty for a certain population. What was the response of regional boards to bed norms? Evidence from the Leeds Region indicates that, while there was often disagreement with the Ministry's guidance, for the most part the Ministry insisted on the Leeds Board following national norms rather than its own preferred standards. This came out quite clearly in 1962 when the Board raised objections to the norms proposed for mental illness, mental handicap and geriatric services in the Hospital Plan, in each case preferring to plan on the basis of higher norms. The Ministry overruled the Board, as it had done on previous occasions, and insisted that planning should proceed on the basis of national guidelines.

However, the actual impact, in terms of levels of service provision, was uneven: the number of mental illness beds was reduced, but at a slower rate than envisaged; the number of mental handicap beds remained the same, even though a small reduction was required according to Ministry norms; and the number of geriatric beds remained the same, even though a reduction from 1.7 beds per thousand population to 1.4 beds per thousand population was required. Short of cutting off funds for these services, which as far as is known was never contemplated as a serious option, and indeed would have been contrary to the policy of giving priority to long-stay services which emerged in the late 1960s, it is difficult to see how the central department could ensure compliance with these norms. Certainly, the department lacked a capacity for sustained analysis and review of the policies it was pursuing and the way in which they were being implemented. Brown makes a similar point, noting that the Ministry's 'headquarters staff was very small and was, moreover, preoccupied with routine and parliamentary business, with little scope for policy-making and review'.[19] This did not change radically until the 1972 reorganisation of DHSS, which created new divisions within the headquarters organisation responsible for liaising with field authorities (see Chapter 1).

Potentially much more important than either circulars or norms was the power of direction conferred on the Minister by the NHS Act, 1946. An interesting example of the use of this power arose in the Leeds Region in 1956, involving an anaesthetist employed by the Board as a senior hospital medical officer.[20] During a review of gradings the anaesthetist was awarded consultant status and subsequently applied for her post to be upgraded to that of consultant. This the Board refused to do, arguing that an additional consultant post was not justified in the area in which the doctor worked. With assistance from the British Medical Association, the anaesthetist then submitted an appeal to the Regional Appeals Committee of the Whitley Council, which decided in her favour. At this point the Board sought counsel's opinion on the effect of the decision. The Board believed that if it accepted the Appeals Committee's decision it would be acting *ultra vires* since statutory regulations required consultant appointments to be made only after advertisement. Moreover, the Board felt an important point of principle was involved in that it alone had control over its establishment. Counsel supported the Board, stating that the Appeals Committee's decision was not binding, but adding that the Minister could nevertheless direct the Board to implement the decision under Section 12 of the NHS Act. The Board's solicitors added that any such direction

> would constitute a serious inroad into the rights and obligations of the Board to administer services within their area, and in our opinion the Minister ought not lightly to make any such direction, as in effect he would be allowing the BMA to settle the establishment for specialists in the area.

On receiving this advice the Board decided not to implement the decision, and subsequently the Minister directed the Board to do so.

It should be noted that this was an exceptional case. Indeed, it was the only occasion when the power of direction was invoked against the Leeds Board. The case nevertheless illustrates that control lay ultimately at the centre, and indicates the power of the medical profession, a point which is developed later.

Granted that this was an exceptional case, on the whole relations between boards and the department were amicable and conflict-free. These good relations were fostered by the continuous dialogue which took place through the medium of meetings between regional members and officers and Ministers and department officials; the presence in regions of the Ministry's principal regional officers; bilateral policy review meetings; and discussions between departmental and board officials on particular projects and services. These contacts enabled the department to find out what was happening in the regions and to inform boards of the way thinking was developing at the centre. In turn, boards notified the department of problems they were experiencing, and initiatives they were making. At this level the relationship was essentially one of mutual adjustment and influence and of working together.

We have seen that during Enoch Powell's term of office the Ministry and boards worked particularly closely together in preparing and implementing the Hospital Plan. Boards were keen to take advantage of the additional money which had become available for hospital building and were only too willing to move in step with the centre. The relationship was not so much one of control, but of broad agreement between centre and periphery on the direction in which the Service should be developing. In contrast, Richard Crossman wanted boards to reallocate resources in a way they considered impossible. Understandably frustrated at his inability to move boards in the direction he wanted, it was not surprising that Crossman concluded that the centre was weak and boards were strong. An additional factor behind the different perceptions of Powell and Crossman was the changing economic and financial climate. This meant that the period of rapid expansion in the early 1960s which lay behind the Hospital Plan had given way to a concern with rising costs at the end of the decade, making it harder to achieve the shift of resources Crossman was seeking. As Crossman himself noted in relation to the geographical distribution of funds, it is more difficult to pursue a Robin Hood policy of robbing the rich to help the poor at a time of limited growth.[21] This helps explain the conflicting views of Powell and Crossman.

Overall, then, the evidence suggests that, when there was agreement at board level with departmental policy, the centre and regions moved together. On the other hand, when there was disagreement the centre had to find alternative means of imposing its will. In extreme cases the means might be the power of direction, but at other times new policy instruments, such as earmarking funds, had to be found. As the official view of department/board relations states, the department did control total expenditure, issue guidance on policy and priorities, and approve key expenditure decisions like major building projects. Except in the early years of the NHS, the centre generally avoided detailed interference in local management. What this indicates is that the balance between the department and boards varied according to what the centre was attempting to achieve, changed over time, and differed between areas of service provision.

Where did this leave HMCs? Since it would have been too great a task for the central department to deal individually with nearly 400 HMCs, the department sought to control and influence HMCs through regional boards. However, as early as March 1948 the Ministry by-passed boards by issuing a circular direct to HMCs, and at a meeting with Ministry officials board chairmen protested at what they saw as unwarranted interference in their supervisory functions. Following a discussion, the chairman of the Leeds Board reported that:

> the chairmen were of opinion that the discussion showed that there was no intention to impair the responsibility of the regional boards or to interfere with the day-to-day responsibility of management committees, and there was a general feeling that matters should now be allowed to work themselves out in practice in a spirit of mutual understanding and sympathy.

Yet circulars continued to be sent to HMCs as well as boards, and the uncertainty of relationships was reflected in the Guillebaud Committee's conclusion that:

> Regional Hospital Boards should be told, and Hospital Management Committees should accept, that the Regional Boards are responsible for exercising a general oversight and supervision over the administration of the hospital service in their Regions. It is a corollary of this recommendation that the Ministry should leave the task of supervising the Hospital Management Committees to the Regional Boards and should not undertake this task over the heads of the Boards.[22]

We have noted earlier how the supervisory powers of boards were increased from the mid 1950s onwards. Arguably, this process went too far, for the first green paper on NHS reorganisation, published in 1968, maintained that:

> the interest which Regional Hospital Boards have increasingly taken in the performance of management functions by Hospital Management Committees, though not outside their statutory powers, may go beyond what was envisaged when the structure was established. Their primary task as orginally conceived was planning and co-ordinating development; their intervention in matters of management has grown out of their responsibility for allocating financial resources, but is sometimes unwelcome. Confused responsibilities tend to create unsatisfactory relationships.[23]

The Leeds Board disputed the implied criticism in this statement, and it does seem that the statement was based more on the need to justify the abolition of the regional tier in the NHS than on a thorough analysis of administrative relationships. Certainly, the members and officers from the Board and HMCs interviewed during the research argued that relationships in the Leeds Region were good, and the high degree of overlapping membership which existed contributed to this. Regular meetings were also held between the chairman and senior officers of the Board and their HMC counterparts. Documentary evidence reveals no major disputes, and in some cases it demonstrates the reverse: thus in April 1951, in announcing that the Board had decided to delegate to HMCs responsibility for deciding how the cuts made in the estimates should be allocated, the chairman of the Finance Committee said the Board was prepared to entrust this task to HMCs in order to preserve 'the spirit of mutual confidence which has been built up in the last three years on the solid basis of the full appreciation of respective functions'.

Good relations did not, however, mean that management committees simply accepted Board, or indeed Ministry, policy. We have noted in this chapter that HMCs objected to Crossman's request that funds be diverted to long-stay services from within existing budgets, and elsewhere in the book we have drawn attention to other examples of local resistance to regional and national policy. More often than not, this resistance stemmed from group medical advisory committees which tended to exercise a strong influence over HMCs, and the significance of the medical profession in the structure of administrative control is discussed below. Faced with local resistance, the Board had to proceed by means of persuasion and influence rather than by direction. As far as we could discover, the ultimate sanction of not reappointing HMC members because of conflict over policy was never used by the Board. However, there was one instance when the Board, under strong pressure from DHSS, did not reappoint an HMC chairman, apparently because of the Secretary of State's displeasure at the way an incident at a long-stay hospital had been handled. Far more frequent were the cases when HMC chairmen and members were not reappointed because of the Board's policy of rationalising the management committee structure and reducing the number of committee members. These cases demonstrated that the destinies of HMCs were, in a literal sense, in the control of the Board, but this power was not used as a sanction. Overall, then, HMCs stood in much the same relationship to the Board as did the latter to the central department: they exercised their powers within the broad constraints imposed by regionally-allocated budgets, and by regional and national policy decisions.

A comparison with local government

A contrast can be drawn between the department's relationship with local authorities and its relationship with regional boards. This contrast can be illustrated by differences between the Hospital Plan and the equivalent plan for local authorities, Health and Welfare: The Development of Community Care. While the former was a national plan drawn up in accordance with guidelines laid down by the Ministry, the latter was very much a collection of the individual plans of local authorities throughout the country in which national guidelines had had much less impact. This was evident from the wide variations in the level of services which local authorities were planning to provide. To use the terminology of J. A. G. Griffith, if the Ministry's attitude to local authorities were 'laissez-faire', then its attitude to hospital authorities was 'promotional'.[24] This interpretation is supported by the DHSS evidence to the Public Expenditure Committee referred to earlier. Thus the balance between central control and local autonomy was closer to the centre in the hospital service than in local government.

How can this be explained? Self has listed the three conditions which maximise the autonomy of an agency, and it is illuminating to apply these to local government and regional hospital boards. The three conditions are: a real abnegation of governmental policy control; the existence of a task which can be treated in relative isolation from the rest of government; and the availability of an independent and adequate source of revenue.[25] Looking at local government first, governmental policy control has been steadily increasing as a result of growing political demands for greater uniformity in service provision, while the financial independence of local government has been progressively declining as government grants have taken up a higher proportion of local government expenditure. Moreover, many of local government's functions are not self-contained, personal social services being an obvious example: hence the move towards centralization noted by the Layfield Committee and others.[26] As far as the hospital service is concerned, at no time has any of the three conditions obtained. The degree of governmental policy control has, however, varied, and this accounts for the changing balance of the relationship over time.

Self goes on to argue that a further condition of agency independence is the absence of any powerful group of clients or suppliers who can supplement their control for that of the withdrawing government. While no such group is evident in local government, the medical profession is an obvious candidate in the hospital service, and the extent of medical influence in the NHS, sometimes held to amount to syndicalism, is a familiar theme. Richard Crossman, for instance, as well as maintaining that boards were strong, contended that the hospital service was 'consultant dominated'.[27] Similarly, in evidence to the Public Expenditure Committee, DHSS stated that 'the existence of clinical freedom substantially reduces the ability of the central authorities to determine objectives and priorities and to control individual facets of expenditure'.[28] Klein has argued that it was precisely this freedom and the influence exerted by the profession on boards and through advisory committees that prevented Crossman and other Ministers from diverting resources to long-stay services.[29]

What this suggests is that, in addition to examining the relationship between boards and the department, the influence of the profession at both levels needs to be studied, as does the part played by the profession in conflicts between the two. Through the BMA and membership of working parties, advisory committees and the like at national level the profession does undoubtedly exercise power. To return to an earlier example, increasing central control of hospital doctor appointments was increasing central *medical* control, as the profession dominated both the Central Manpower Committee, and its forerunner, the Advisory Committee on Consultant Establishments. As a number of studies have shown, on issues like staffing and remuneration, and on policies like health service reorganisation, doctors have exerted considerable influence at the national level.

A similar situation existed at regional board level, where medical representation was around 25 per cent and where an extensive system of medical advisory committees operated. Again, in the single case in which the Ministry used the power of direction over the Leeds Board, the influence of the profession was readily apparent. Not only did the centre come down in favour of the aggrieved doctor, but also the Board's solicitors' statement (that to make the direction 'would be allowing the BMA to settle the establishment for specialists in the area') indicated the real source of power in this case.

Many other examples of professional influence have been cited in this book, and, at the risk of repetition, it is worth mentioning again issues like resistance to the bed reallocation plans put forward by the Board in the 1950s; the opposition of psychiatrists to the designation of secure units for the mentally ill; and the rejection by paediatricians of proposals for developing children's hospitals services in Leeds. All of these examples illustrate the importance of professional control as well as administrative control in the NHS.

Conclusion

The preceding discussion and analysis have drawn out some of the complexities of centre–periphery relationships in the hospital service between 1948 and 1974. As far as the main theme of the chapter – central department/regional board relations – is concerned, it has been suggested that the strong central control established immediately after the formation of the NHS was prompted by Treasury concern with escalating costs, and that this control was relaxed during the 1950s but increased again at the end of the 1960s, principally because of the desire by DHSS to shift resources between services (and later regions), but also partly because of rising costs. The capacity of the central department to ensure that its policies were implemented was limited, however, even though a variety of means of control – financial, legal, advisory – were available. Persuasion and influence were the main currency in which the department dealt with boards, and its style became more promotional and interventionist as the 1960s progressed. But while boards were rather more tightly controlled than local health authorities, they still had considerable autonomy to pursue their own policies. Much the same applied to HMCs, which the central department sought to control through boards. The relationship between boards and management committees was similar to the relationship between the central department and boards, with persuasion being the main means of supervision and control. If management committees were not inclined to follow regional or national policy, then there was little boards could do except cajole, advise and encourage. And it was particularly at HMC level that professional influence was strong. The position of the medical profession in the structure of administrative control was important in sometimes frustrating the achievement of national and regional policies, and it was this factor as much as any other which inhibited the development of a centralised service. It is also a warning against drawing simple central control or regional autonomy conclusions in a service as politically complex as the NHS.

9

Lessons and Conclusions

In this chapter we move out from the specific field of the Leeds Regional Hospital Board and discuss the general lessons of the study both for the NHS and for students of policy-making and implementation. The chapter does not provide a comprehensive summary of our findings as this would be repetitive and unhelpful. Rather, we have taken the opportunity to address some of the broader questions raised by our study, taking it for granted that readers will be familiar with the detail of the earlier chapters.

Other writers have drawn up a balance sheet for the NHS, comparing achievements with intentions. Both Brown and Watkin do this, and the conclusion they reach is that the credits outweigh the debits: that, while there are some remaining distortions and deficiencies in health services, on the whole the NHS represents good value for money.[1] Money is in fact the key to any assessment of the NHS, since it is by examining the way in which money is allocated and spent that it is possible to judge what kind of service is being provided.

In the early years of the NHS the Beveridge assumption that expenditure would decline when the backlog of ill-health was reduced was exposed as a fallacy. Expenditure then and later continued to increase, from £433 million in 1949 to £3900 million in 1974. Over the same period NHS expenditure as a proportion of GDP increased from 3.95 per cent to 5.3 per cent. One of the reasons for these increases was that advances in medical technology made possible a whole new range of interventions, like hip replacements and renal dialysis. At the same time additional services like family planning and abortion were made generally available. Despite the upward spiral of expenditure, there was always a demand for more money, particularly from professional interests. Enoch Powell, Minister of Health from 1960 to 1963, noted 'the continual, deafening chorus of complaint which rises day and night from every part'[2] of the NHS, and warnings of imminent crisis and collapse unless additional funds were found became a common characteristic. International comparisons lent some justification to the claim for more resources. Whereas in 1972 the United Kingdom was spending 5.2 per cent of GNP on health care, the United States was spending 7.7 per cent and France 5.6 per cent. Yet there was little evidence that more money brought better results. As one study concluded: 'Based on such international data as are available . . . the NHS seems to perform reasonably and to provide good value for money'.[3] Indeed, a state medical service with a limited private sector had, in the eyes of some observers, an advantage precisely because it was able to control costs.[4]

By the early 1970s the knowledge that there would never be enough money to meet all demands on the health service led to a closer examination of how existing funds were being used. In particular there was a concern that doctors, as major resource controllers, were neither as effective nor as efficient as they might be. There was evidence, for example, that heart attack patients were just as likely to recover at home as in an expensive coronary care unit. Also, there were wide variations among doctors in the time they kept patients with similar conditions in hospital. Moreover, some interventions were entirely unproven in their effectiveness. The assault was led by Cochrane,[5] an epidemiologist, closely followed by health economists[6] and politicians.[7] This unholy trinity of corporate rationalisers represented a serious challenge to medical autonomy and dominance. At the same time, the cultural critique of medical sociologists,[8] and, more idiosyncratically, of Ivan Illich,[9] questioned the whole basis of professional involvement in health.

The reverberations in the NHS were expressed in the concern to give greater priority to prevention and care rather than cure; to achieve a more equitable geographical distribution of funds and manpower; and to develop closer links both between the different parts of the NHS and between health services and other related services. Despite a policy commitment to these aims, the effect on the ground was often less than impressive. The development of community care for the mentally ill was a case in point: hence the 1974 reorganisation, with its promise of more efficient management, an integrated health service, and better contacts with local authority services.

While it is probably too early to make a proper assessment of the impact of reorganisation, there is an emerging consensus that the hoped for benefits have not been realised. Brown's study of Humberside (part of which was in the Leeds Region) has noted that structural change of the kind carried out in 1974 has serious drawbacks. Brown's principal conclusions are that reorganisation involves heavy costs in terms of disturbance, delay and uncertainty; most of the costs arise from structural changes; structural changes increase permanent running costs; and reorganisation generates over-optimism about the net advantages to be gained.[10]

But what of the place of the regional tier in the administrative structure? Here Brown echoes Godber in arguing that, 'A regional tier of some sort is almost indispensable for NHS administration in England: administration from London would be too remote'.[11] What reasons can be advanced in support of this argument? The main factor in favour of a regional authority is the need for a body close enough to the ground to possess knowledge of local conditions and services, and yet sufficiently detached to be able to make broad judgements about priorities. In other words, the need for some form of regional planning is the principal justification for a regional tier. Our own study provides ample evidence to support this view. Among the benefits to accrue from the planning activities of the Leeds RHB were a rationalised and co-ordinated policy for infectious diseases hospitals; significant improvements in hospital services in those areas which in 1948 were identified as in greatest need; much improved hospital provision for the elderly, particularly insofar as acute units in general hospitals and medical staffing levels were concerned; and a more equitable distribution of senior medical staff. Of course, the Board's history is not just a story of one long path of advancement, and we have given plenty of examples of national and regional policy goals which were not implemented. Nevertheless, it can be claimed with some justification that the strategic planning role exercised at regional level was behind many of the advances made in the hospital service in the first phase of the NHS.

The interposition of regional hospital boards between the central department and hospital management committees also meant there was a certain loss of control by the central department. We hope to have shown that boards were not simply the Minister's agents, unthinkingly applying national policies to their areas. Rather, boards had an independent policy-making role, even if they were not the 'independent realms'[12] which Richard Crossman claimed. Inevitably, this meant that there were occasions when boards disagreed with national policies and priorities and pursued their own preferences instead. When this happened there was little the Department could do except argue, cajole and persuade: hence the importance of the NHS Planning System introduced in 1976, which was in part an attempt to secure greater conformity of local services with national policies.

The Planning System can be seen as the process change, the change in the way things get done and decisions are taken, to accompany the 1974 structural change in the NHS. The aims of the System are to achieve the kinds of switch in resources from hospital to community services and from acute to long-stay services that were so difficult to achieve before reorganisation. In design the System is an attempt to introduce rational and comprehensive planning into the NHS: planners are expected to define their aims, review existing services, select among options according to resource availability, implement the chosen options, monitor and evaluate results, and so on.[13] The intention is that planning by decibels – 'he who shouts the loudest gets the most'[14] – will be replaced by a rational approach in which the emphasis is on arguments buttressed by information, and the implementation of agreed policies.

Yet, although great store has been set by the System, there are already signs that local pressures are causing a reversal of national priorities. The document with which the System was launched in 1976, *Priorities for Health and Personal Social Services in England*, contained, among other things, a commitment to cut expenditure on acute services and on hospital maternity services. Both commitments have subsequently been reversed.[15] What this suggests is that neither structural change nor process change can overcome the power of professionals at the local level. As Towell has argued:

In the case of NHS reorganisation, the basic objectives were to encourage the more rational, effective and integrated use of resources in providing improved health care for the people. This was to be achieved through changes in organisation structure, notably through unifying the administration of hitherto separate services, and in management processes relating particularly to planning, consultation and multi-disciplinary team decision-making . . . left less than fully stated were the changes in power relationships required in order to achieve any radical impact in the prevailing distribution of resources, both between different types of health provision and between different parts of the country.[16]

It is at this point that it may be appropriate to examine the nature of these power relationships by considering what lessons our study holds for students of health policy-making and implementation.

Policy and power in the health service

In the Introduction we mentioned that the analysis of policy is concerned with both the analysis of policy processes and the analysis of the distribution of power. In terms of policy processes, what we have found is that a number of different individuals, groups and interests were involved in policy-making in the Leeds RHB, that none of these interests had the power to impose its will on all of the others, that consequently decision-making took the form of bargaining in a system of bureaucratic politics, and that the resultant was usually a small change in the *status quo*. What is more, the political and organisational complexity of the decision-making environment meant that it was sometimes difficult to achieve any kind of change; or, as we argued in Chapter 6, 'in policy systems where there are many different interests and where power is not concentrated in an individual or group, it is easier to prevent change than to achieve it. Successful policy promotion in such systems is dependent on the winning of a coalition of support by an active individual or interest.'

Of course, the dominant incrementalist mode was sometimes departed from, and we have drawn attention to aspects of rationality and comprehensiveness in the planning activities undertaken by the Leeds Board, as well as occasional radical shifts in service provision. Indeed, as we argued above, it was when these aspects were in the ascendant that the case for a regional tier was most clear. What tended to frustrate the pursuit of more rational policies was the strength of medical interests. To quote again from an earlier chapter: 'in the NHS the existence of powerful professional interests at the operational level is likely to be the main obstacle to the implementation of agreed policies'. A number of factors contributed to the power of the medical profession: their membership of RHBs and

HMCs; their influence through medical advisory committees; their position as direct service providers; and the deference accorded to medical views and opinions. And, since the profession was in a dominant position, small changes helped maintain this dominance.

Thus, while policy processes may have been incremental, plural and characterised by bargaining and compromise, the distribution of power was weighed heavily in favour of the professional monopolisers. Although the corporate rationalisers at Board level won some battles, very often they did not pursue their challenge to medical dominance. As Brown has commented about the reorganised NHS: 'The danger is that strategic intentions will, as in the past, be compromised by a succession of *ad hoc* incrementalist managerial decisions at the periphery'.[17] A further point to note is that within the medical profession power was unevenly distributed. All of our evidence indicates that the main beneficiaries were those in acute specialties, and senior medical staff rather than junior. By 1974 there were some signs that this was beginning to change, and that within the profession the interests of junior doctors were being actively articulated and asserted. At the same time, there were attempts to give greater priority to the Cinderella services by strengthening the role of corporate rationalisers, through the Planning System and the new specialty of community medicine; and to bolster the voice of the community through community health councils.

Equally significant, the hitherto muted voice of health service ancillary workers became a factor to be reckoned with for the first time. Ancillary workers and the trade unions which represent them have not figured prominently in this study, precisely because their position in the NHS power structure did not become apparent until 1973. It was in that year that a series of strikes over wage negotiations marked an end to 'the belief that the Health Service's labour relations were qualitatively different from those of industry'.[18] Subsequent union involvement in, and industrial action on, other issues like pay beds and hospital closures was a further reminder that the corporate rationalisers and the community population were not the only interests to challenge the professional monopolisers. Indeed, the growth of union activity suggests the need to add a fourth category – perhaps labelled 'worker organisation' – to the other three suggested by Alford.[19]

Lessons for the study of policy

As well as seeking to illuminate various aspects of health services and
health policy, this study has sought to examine the experiences of the
Leeds RHB from a policy analysis perspective. Policy analysis is a
developing field of study, and it draws its inspiration from a number
of different disciplines. Wildavsky has maintained that 'the technical
base of policy analysis is weak,'[20] a judgement supported by the
range of ideas and concepts used in this study. There is very little in
the way of a core body of work which can be identified, and the
literature used here, drawn more from political science than any other
discipline, is as much a reflection of the author's own biases as a
commentary on the state of the art of policy analysis.

By way of conclusion, then, what lessons are there for those who
seek to study policy? First, we have found the vocabulary of decision
theory – incrementalism, mixed scanning and rational comprehensiveness – to be helpful in describing the Board's approach
to policy-making. Moreover, in looking at policy processes we have
noted the importance of focusing on the interactions between
decision makers. Policy-making in the Leeds RHB, insofar as it can be
distinguished from policy implementation, typically took place in the
interstices of the Board's committee system and in negotiations
between officers, and we have discussed some of the struggles which
resulted. Again, an examination of the central government response
to the Ely report, where, unusually, data are available through the
Crossman Diaries, has pointed to the bargaining which occurred
between politicians, civil servants and other interests. There is a
lesson here for prospective studies: that there is a need to get inside
'the black box' and understand more closely the system of bargaining, compromise and negotiation which occurs between decision
makers. Problems of gaining access should not be underestimated,
but the rewards to be reaped are high, as studies by Heclo and
Wildavsky and Edwards and Batley have shown[21].

Secondly, in examining the distribution of power in the health
policy system, Alford's discussion of professional monopolisers,
corporate rationalisers and the community population has been
found the most useful way of conceptualising the different interests
involved. We agree with Alford that the conflicts between these
interests are not best seen as a struggle between pressure groups in a
pluralist system. Rather, the important point to note is that the

dominant interests – the professional monopolisers – are systematically benefited by the *status quo*. This is much closer to élite theory's explanation of power than that of pluralist theory. As Alford goes on to argue, the fact that there is a broad consensus about health services and health policy reinforces the position of the medical profession, and:

> the existence of a network of political, legal and economic institutions which guarantees that certain dominant interests will be served comes to be taken for granted as legitimate, as the only possible way in which these health services can be provided.[22]

One of the consequences for the study of policy is the need to look in more detail at how this consensus is created and maintained. In turn, this may provide a link between analysis of the policy process and analysis of the distribution of power. It is self-evident that policy is not made and unmade in a value vacuum, and that actors' beliefs, attitudes and perceptions influence how they behave. The policy analysis literature has paid little attention to these issues, and the origin of actors' values and beliefs and their effect on policy-making and implementation is less than clear.

An exception is Vickers' discussion of 'appreciative system', which he defines as 'a set of readiness to distinguish some aspects of the situation rather than others and to classify and value these in this way rather than that'.[23] The appreciative system helps determine how situations are perceived, and as such acts as an interpretative screen. Vickers' work lies behind Young's concept, 'assumptive worlds',[24] which can be seen to be organised hierarchically as ideology, attitudes and opinion. As Young and Mills argue in a later paper:

> We might think here of ideology as a generalised, symbolic and taken-for-granted representation of the world we live in; of mediating 'values' and beliefs as middle range constructs for managing the world presented to us; and of opinions as the circumstantial and specific responses to the everyday world we encounter.[25]

Young and Mills maintain that:

> an understanding of the assumptive worlds of government actors is

essential to successful policy analysis, for it enables us to interpret events in the light of the meanings which the actors involved ascribe to their own actions, rather than interpret these actions in terms of postulated interests, motives or goals.[26]

The need, then, is to move towards more interpretative approaches, and to examine how far and in what way actors' values are socially constructed. There are a number of issues for research here, including the identification of assumptive worlds, and the specification of the interaction between assumptive worlds and dominant belief systems on the one hand, and assumptive worlds and problem definition in the policy process on the other hand. Also, the relationship between belief systems and the power structure has been insufficiently articulated.

To give a concrete example of some of these issues, one of the most interesting cases to emerge from this study was the handling of acute hospital admissions in Leeds, described in Chapter 6. On the basis of the available data, we have argued that certain groups in the medical profession, because of their dominant position in the power structure, were able to define the acute admissions' problem in a way that best suited their interests. What is less clear is how these groups – that is, those representing the interests of the teaching hospital and acute specialties – were able to use their dominance to shape policy-makers' values, preferences and beliefs. One explanation would be that as powerful interests they established the primacy of teaching and research, and that this influenced policy-makers to the extent that their values led them to define the problem as to how to create a better teaching hospital service. Alternative explanations and definitions were ignored or not even perceived because they ranked low in the prevalent system of values and beliefs. There are clearly links here with the literature on power, in particular Lukes' discussion of the third dimension of power. Lukes' point that power can be exercised in the absence of conflict and against the interests of those excluded from decision-making processes would appear to be applicable to this case. In Lukes' terminology, the 'relevant counterfactual'[27] which supports this interpretation was the later redefinition of the problem as how to provide an effective geriatric service.

In the absence of information about policy-makers' values and perceptions, these can only be speculations, but this case suggests a bundle of researchable issues, any one of which would provide a fruitful area for further work. To conclude, then, there are many gaps in our knowledge, and this is a challenge to the student of policy. What we hope to have shown is that the NHS, as well as being 'a game reserve for political scientists interested in analysing the role of pressure groups',[28] is also an arena where some of these wider policy questions can be pursued.

Notes and References

Introduction

1. Birmingham RHB, *Birmingham RHB 1947–1966* (Birmingham: Arthur Thomson House, 1966); M. Ryan, *The Welsh Hospital Board* (Cardiff, not dated).
2. 'A region reports', *The Hospital*, vol. 62 [a] (September 1966) p. 417.
3. A. Lindsey, *Socialised Medicine in England and Wales* (Chapel Hill: University of North Carolina Press, 1962).
4. R. Stevens, *Medical Practice in Modern England* (New Haven: Yale University Press, 1966).
5. R. G. S. Brown, *The Changing National Health Service* (London: Routledge and Kegan Paul, 1973); G. Forsyth, *Doctors and State Medicine* (London: Pitman, 1971); B. Watkin, *The National Health Service: The First Phase* (London: George Allen and Unwin, 1978); B. Abel-Smith, *National Health Service: The first thirty years* (London: HMSO, 1978).
6. G. Godber, *The Health Service: Past, Present and Future* (London: Athlone Press, 1975); R. H. S. Crossman, *A Politician's View of Health Service Planning* (University of Glasgow, 1972), and *The Diaries of a Cabinet Minister*, vol. 3 (London: Hamish Hamilton and Jonathan Cape, 1977); D. Owen, *In Sickness and In Health* (London: Quartet, 1976).
7. R. Klein, 'Policy problems and policy perceptions in the National Health Service', *Policy and Politics*, vol. 2 [3] (1974) p. 219.
8. R. G. S. Brown, *The Management of Welfare* (London: Fontana, 1975) p. 51.
9. H. Eckstein, *Pressure Group Politics* (London: Allen and Unwin, 1960).
10. R. A. Dahl, *Who Governs?* (New Haven: Yale University Press, 1961); P. Bachrach and M. S. Baratz, *Power and Poverty* (New York: Oxford University Press, 1970).
11. I. Gordon, J. Lewis and K. Young, 'Perspectives on policy analysis', *Public Administration Bulletin*, December 1977.
12. G. T. Allison, *Essence of Decision* (Boston: Little Brown, 1971).
13. R. Klein, 'Policy problems', and 'Policy making in the National Health

Service', *Political Studies*, vol. 22 [1] (March 1974).

14. H. Heclo, *Modern Social Politics in Britain and Sweden* (New Haven: Yale University Press, 1974).
15. J. Higgins, *The Poverty Business* (Oxford: Basil Blackwell, 1978).
16. P. Hall, H. Land, R. Parker and A. Webb, *Change, Choice and Conflict in Social Policy* (London: Heinemann, 1975).
17. C. J. Ham, 'Approaches to the study of social policy making', *Policy and Politics*, vol. 8, no. 1 (January 1980).
18. This committee was split into a Finance Committee and a General Purposes Committee between 1950 and 1967, and for this period research effort was directed to the latter.
19. This Committee resulted from the merger of the Mental Health Committee and the Geriatrics Committee in 1961. Before that date the minutes of both committees were examined in detail.
20. For a discussion of this, see Bachrach and Baratz, *Power and Poverty*.
21. For example, J. Dearlove, *The Politics of Policy in Local Government* (London: Cambridge University Press, 1973).
22. R. H. S. Crossman, *The Diaries of a Cabinet Minister*, vol. 1, *Minister of Housing, 1964–1966* (London: Hamilton and Cape, 1975) pp. 103–4.
23. J. Carrier and I. Kendall, 'The development of welfare states: The production of plausible accounts', *Journal of Social Policy*, vol. 6 [3] p. 290.
24. Allison, *Essence of Decision*.
25. H. Heclo and A. Wildavsky, *The Private Government of Public Money* (London: Macmillan, 1974).
26. See notes, 14, 15 and 16.
27. For example, Heclo in *Modern Social Politics*.
28. Allison, *Essence of Decision*.

Chapter 1

1. B. Abel-Smith, *The Hospitals 1800–1948* (London: Heinemann, 1964) p. 491.
2. Ibid.
3. R. M. Titmuss, *Problems of Social Policy* (London: HMSO, 1950) p. 460.
4. The surveys were summarised in Nuffield Provincial Hospitals Trust, *The Hospital Surveys: The Domesday Book of the Hospital Service* (London: Oxford University Press, 1946).
5. H. Eason, R. V. Clark, and W. H. Harper, *Hospital Survey: The Hospital Services of the Yorkshire Area* (London: HMSO, 1945).
6. Ibid., p. 19.
7. Ibid., p. 20. In this context 'pure' specialist refers to those not engaged in general practice.
8. Ibid., p. 40.
9. Ibid., p. 57.
10. See, for example, Abel-Smith, *The Hospitals*, p. 408; Titmuss, *Problems of Social Policy*, p. 66; and Nuffield Provincial Hospitals Trust, *The Hospital Surveys*, pp. 13–15.

11. H. Eckstein, *The English Health Service* (Cambridge, Mass: Harvard University Press, 1958), pp. 62–3.
12. Eason, Clark and Harper, *Hospital Survey*, p. 21.
13. Ibid., p. 42.
14. Ibid., p. 88.
15. Nuffield Provincial Hospitals Trust, *The Hospital Surveys*, p. 15.
16. Eason. Clark and Harper, *Hospital Survey*, p. 23.
17. Abel-Smith, *The Hospitals*, p. 440.
18. *A National Health Service*, Cmd. 6502 (London: HMSO, 1944).
19. A. J. Willcocks, *The Creation of the National Health Service* (London: Routledge and Kegan Paul, 1967) p. 68.
20. Abel-Smith, *The Hospitals*, p. 471.
21. Willcocks, *The Creation of the National Health Service*, p. 63.
22. Hansard, vol. 422, cols. 49–50.
23. Ibid.
24. This remark is widely attributed to Bevan, although I have not been able to find the source. Julian Tudor Hart quotes the phrase 'choked their mouths with gold' as an alternative. See 'Bevan and the Doctors', *Lancet*, 1973 vol. 2, pp. 1196–7. His source is a personal communication with Brian Abel-Smith.
25. Ministry of Health, Circular RHB(47)1.
26. Ministry of Health, Circular RHB(48)2.
27. Ministry of Health, Circular RHB(47)1.
28. Ibid.
29. A Bevan, *In Place of Fear* (London: MacGibbon and Kee, 1961) new edition, pp. 99–100.
30. Ibid., pp. 114–15.
31. *Report of the Committee of Enquiry into the Cost of the National Health Service*, Cmd. 9663 (London: HMSO, 1956).
32. B. Abel-Smith and R. M. Titmuss, *The Cost of the National Health Service* (Cambridge: Cambridge University Press, 1956).
33. *Report of the Committee of Enquiry*, p. 57.
34. Ibid.
35. Acton Society Trust, *Hospitals and the State*, i. *Background and Blueprint*, 1955; ii. *Impact of the Change*, 1956; iii. *Hospital Management Committees*, 1957; iv. *Regional Hospital Boards*, 1957; v. *The Central Control of the Service*, 1957; vi. *Creative Leadership in a State Service*, 1959.
36. Eckstein, *The English Health Service*, pp. 259–60.
37. L. Abel and W. Lewin, 'Report on hospital building', *British Medical Journal Supplement*, 4 April 1959, pp. 109–14.
38. B. Davies, *Social Needs and Resources in Local Services* (London: Michael Joseph, 1968) p. 206.
39. D. S. Lees, *Health Through Choice* (London: Institute of Economic Affairs, 1961).
40. *A Review of the Medical Services in Great Britain* (London: Social Assay, 1962) p. 1.
41. Ibid., p. 14.

42. Ibid., p. 20.
43. *The Administrative Structure of the Medical and Related Services in England and Wales* (London: HMSO, 1968) pp. 9–10.
44. *Report of the Committee of Enquiry into Allegations of Ill-Treatment of Patients and other irregularities at the Ely Hospital, Cardiff*, Cmnd. 3975 (London: HMSO, 1969).
45. *Administrative Practice of Hospital Boards in Scotland* (Edinburgh: HMSO, 1966); *First Report of the Joint Working Party on the Organisation of Medical Work in Hospitals* (London: HMSO, 1967): second and third reports were published in 1972 and 1974; *Report of the Committee on Senior Nursing Staff Structure* (London: HMSO, 1966).
46. *The Future Structure of the National Health Service* (London: HMSO, 1970).
47. *National Health Service Reorganisation: Consultative Document* (London: DHSS, 1971) p. 6.
48. Ibid., p. 9.
49. This study, which was carried out with the assistance of the management consultants, McKinsey's, and the Health Services Organisational Research Unit at Brunel University, was published as *Management Arrangements for the Reorganised NHS* (London: HMSO, 1972) and known as the Grey Book.
50. *Reports* from the Working Party on Collaboration between the NHS and Local Government on its activities (a) to the end of 1972, (b) from January to July 1973, and (c) from July 1973 to April 1974 (all London: HMSO).
51. *NHS Reorganisation in England*, Cmnd. 5055 (London: HMSO, 1972).

Chapter 2

1. This description of the Region is based on that contained in H. Eason, R. V. Clark and W. H. Harper, *Hospital Survey: The Hospital Services of the Yorkshire Area* (London: HMSO, 1945).
2. Richard Crossman, *A Politician's View of Health Service Planning* (University of Glasgow, 1972) p. 23.
3. A distinction was made between the two principal officers, the SAMO and the Secretary, and the chief officers (for example, the Treasurer and Architect). Principal officers were senior to chief officers, but whether they were responsible for the work of chief officers was unclear.
4. *Management Arrangements for the Reorganised National Health Service* (London: HMSO, 1972).
5. *Administrative Practice of Hospital Boards in Scotland* (Edinburgh: HMSO, 1966) pp. 61–2.
6. Action Society Trust, *Hospitals and the State*, iv. *Regional Hospital Boards* (London: 1957) pp. 11–13.
7. Team management by consensus was one of the main planks of NHS reorganisation. It did not always work smoothly. In Solihull, for example, a tribunal of enquiry was set up in 1977 to investigate differences between members of the area management team. See

'Consensus management' *The Hospital*, vol. 73 [7] (July 1977).
8. *Administrative Practice of Hospital Boards in Scotland*, p. 93.
9. Ibid., paras 35–45.
10. *Report of the Ministry of Health for the year ended 31st March 1949* (London: HMSO, 1950) p. 242.
11. K. Jones, *A History of the Mental Health Services* (London: Routledge and Kegan Paul, 1972) p. 278.
12. K. Jones *et al.*, *Opening the Door* (London: Routledge and Kegan Paul, 1975).
13. Acton Society Trust, *Regional Hospital Boards*, p. 6.
14. *Administrative Practice of Hospital Boards in Scotland*, p. 25.
15. R. Klein, 'Policy making in the National Health Service', *Political Studies*, vol. 22 [1] (1974) p. 9.
16. R. G. S. Brown, *Reorganising the National Health Service* (Oxford: Blackwell and Robertson, 1979) pp. vii–viii.

Chapter 3

1. H. Eckstein, *The English Health Service* (Cambridge, Mass: Harvard University Press, 1958) p. 262.
2. The Ministry's figures were published in circular RHB(48)1, which was issued in a slightly revised version in *Ministry of Health: The Development of Consultant Services* (London: HMSO, 1950). We are told that the figures were 'arrived at by the Ministry asking each specialty how many beds they wanted'. See Acton Society Trust, *Hospitals and the State–Regional Hospital Boards* (London: 1957), p. 21. In total they amounted to the provision of some 16 beds per thousand population, compared with actual provision of around 11 beds per thousand in the Leeds Region and England and Wales.
3. A. Etzioni, 'Mixed-scanning: a third approach to decision-making' *Public Administration Review*, 27 (1967).
4. For planning purposes the board divided the Region into 13 district hospital centres, aiming to provide all basic specialties in each of these centres.
5. H. Eason, R. V. Clark and W. H. Harper, *Hospital Survey: The Hospital Services of the Yorkshire Area* (London: HMSO, 1945).
6. This information is based on interviews and correspondence with former Board members and officers, and was reported earlier in K. Barnard and C. Ham, 'The Reallocation of resources: Parallels with past experience' *The Lancet*, 26 June 1976, pp. 1399–1400.
7. C. E. Lindblom, *The Intelligence of Democracy* (New York: The Free Press, 1965). Lindblom is the originator and principal exponent of the incrementalist thesis both as a descriptive and as a prescriptive model of decision-making.
8. *Report of the Committee of Enquiry into the Cost of the National Health Service*, Cmd. 9663 (London: HMSO, 1956) pp. 31–3.
9. *Report of the Ministry of Health for the year ending 31st December 1953*, Cmd. 9321 (London: HMSO, 1954) p. 13.

10. Careful readers will note that this was lower than the acute bed norm of 3.3 beds per thousand put forward in the Hospital Plan (see below). The explanation is that the Board's figure excluded provision for chest diseases, estimated to require 0.775 beds per thousand in 1954.
11. L. A. Abel and W. Lewin, 'Report on hospital building', *British Medical Journal Supplement*, 4 April 1959, pp. 109–14.
12. *A Hospital Plan for England and Wales*, Cmnd. 1604 (London: HMSO, 1962).
13. *Control of Public Expenditure*, Cmnd. 1432 (London: HMSO, 1961).
14. I should like to thank Sir George Godber for discussing with me the development of the Hospital Plan. For an interesting analysis of the Plan as a case-study in policy formation see D. Allen, *Hospital Planning* (London: Pitman Medical, 1979).
15. *Hospital Plan*, p. iii.
16. Ibid., p. 3.
17. Ibid., p. 9.
18. *The Hospital Building Programme*, Cmnd. 3000 (London: HMSO, 1966).
19. Ibid., p. 1.
20. Ibid.
21. Ibid., p. 10.
22. Ibid.
23. Ministry of Health, Circular HM(65)37.
24. This section draws heavily on: *The Hospital*, June 1965, pp. 291–5; *Hospital Building in Great Britain*, Estimates Committee Minutes of Evidence, HC 59–i, 1969/1970 (London: HMSO, 1969); *The Architects' Journal Information Library*, 10 November 1971, pp. 1061–78.
25. The architect for the Eastburn scheme also worked on the 'Best Buy' projects, which were an attempt to plan hospitals as an integral part of the health and welfare services of the communities they served. The two hospitals involved were designed to provide a ratio of only two acute beds per thousand population. See *Hospital Building in Great Britain*, pp. 23–4.
26. *The Functions of the District General Hospital*, Report of the Committee of the Central Health Services Council (London: HMSO, 1969).
27. Ibid.
28. Ibid., p. iv.
29. Ibid., p. v.
30. *Hospital Building in Great Britain*, p. 29. The official was Mr D. Somerville.
31. *Skeffington Committee: People and Planning*, Report of the Committee on Public Participation in Planning (London: HMSO, 1969).
32. A. E. Bennet (ed.), *Community Hospitals: Progress in Development and Evaluation* (Oxford RHB, 1974).
33. DHSS, Circular HSC(IS)75.
34. *Priorities for Health and Personal Social Services in England: A Consultative Document* (London: HMSO, 1976) p. 11.
35. See Chapter 5.
36. *The Hospital Building Programme*, p. 2.

37. K. A. Barnard, 'Health planning – the last of the panaceas' in K. A. Barnard and K. Lee, *NHS Reorganisation: Issues and Prospects* (Leeds: Nuffield Centre for Health Services Studies, University of Leeds, 1974) p. 123.
38. Ibid., p. 122.
39. See M. J. Hill *et al.*, *Implementation and the Central-Local Relationship*, (Bristol: School for Advanced Urban Studies, University of Bristol, 1979); A. King: 'Overload: Problems of governing in the 1970s', *Political Studies*, Vol. 23 (1975); R. Rose, 'Ungovernability: Is there fire behind the smoke?' *Studies in Public Policy*, no. 16 (University of Strathclyde, Glasgow, 1978).
40. R. Alford, *Health Care Politics* (Chicago: University of Chicago, 1975).
41. E. E. Schattschneider, *The Semi-Sovereign People* (New York: Holt Rinehart and Winston, 1960) p. 71.
42. These figures are drawn from Leeds RHB, *Expenditure on Capital Works* (Harrogate, 1974).

Chapter 4

1. *Report of the Inter-Departmental Committee on the Remuneration of Consultants and Specialists*, Cmd. 7420 (London: HMSO, 1948).
2. A. Maynard and A. Walker, *Doctor manpower 1975–2000: Alternative forecasts and their resource implications*, Royal Commission on the National Health Service, Research Paper Number 4 (London: HMSO, 1978) p. 42.
3. Figures are available for 1948 (1468 sessions) and 1960 (2855 sessions) but not for 1952. Between 1948 and 1960 there was a 94 per cent increase in the number of consultant sessions carried out in the Region. In 1952 central control of consultant establishments was introduced, and this had the effect of considerably slowing down the rate of increase of consultants (see note 7 below). In view of this, and having been informed by the Board's officers who were responsible for medical staffing that around 9 WTE consultants (100 sessions) were added to the establishment each year from 1953 onwards, we have calculated that between 1953 and 1960 there was an increase of some 700 consultant sessions. Consequently there must have been an increase of 700 sessions between 1948 and 1952, or 50 per cent of the 1948 total. This is consistent with statistics compiled by the Platt Working Party on the Hospital Medical Staffing Structure (see Reference 17), which show that more than half of the increase in the number of consultants working in the NHS between 1950 and 1959 occurred in the three years 1950–2.
4. Ministry of Health, Circular RHB(50)106.
5. Letter to RHBs, 25 September 1951.
6. G. Godber, *The Health Service: Past, Present and Future* (London: The Athlone Press, 1975) p. 29.
7. The increase in the number of consultants employed in the NHS fell from 8.9 per cent in 1950 to 2.4 per cent in 1953. *Report of the Ministry of*

Health for the year ended 31st December 1953 (London: HMSO, 1954) p. 32.

8. R. Stevens, *Medical Practice in Modern England* (New Haven: Yale University Press, 1966) p. 228.

9. H. Eckstein, *The English Health Service* (Cambridge, Mass: Harvard University Press, 1958) pp. 234–6.

10. M. Ryan, *The Work of the Welsh Hospital Board, 1948–1974* (Cardiff: Welsh Hospital Board, n.d.), p. 17.

11. Stevens, *Medical Practice*, p. 232.

12. To compile these tables, two types of data were required: population figures for different areas and consultant sessions for different areas, each for the years 1948, 1960 and 1972. Gathering these data posed various problems.

The population figures come from reports presented to the Board, and are the populations used by the Board for planning purposes. (In one sense, then, their accuracy does not matter as the figures represent what the Board's officers and members *believed* to be true.) The 1948 figures are derived from the review of services carried out in 1954, and the 1960 figures from the Board's contribution to the Hospital Plan. The 1972 figures are based on the population forecasts contained in the Hospital Plan. Over the whole period the Region's population increased by about 4 per cent, the increases being greatest in Hull and Leeds. There was a slight decline in the Halifax area. Interestingly, the Board's officers believed, not unreasonably, that, because Leeds was a teaching centre it was also a net importer of patients, and the Leeds population was weighted accordingly. Closer examination of hospital statistics after 1974 revealed that Leeds did in fact export patients, mainly to the Wakefield area. If allowances were made for this in the figures presented here, then Leeds would probably come out ahead of Wakefield in the league table.

The main source of the consultant session figures were the Statistical Reviews of Hospital Services in the Leeds Region prepared annually by the Board's officers from 1959 to 1972. The Reviews contain tables setting out the number of sessions in each area for 1948, 1960 and subsequent years up to 1972. The tables *exclude sessions in psychiatry*, which are therefore also excluded from our data. It remained to work out the number of consultant sessions carried out at the United Leeds Hospitals. Figures for 1972 were obtained from the DHSS publication: *Hospital Medical and Dental Staff, 1972.* Figures for 1960 were obtained from staff formerly employed by the Board of Governors of the United Leeds Hospitals (*Hospital Medical and Dental Staff* was published for the first time in 1963, and so could not be used). Figures for 1948 were more problematic, and were derived principally from the annual reports of the United Leeds Hospitals. Careful analysis of these reports, and cross checks with later data, provided a fairly accurate estimate of the *number* of consultants working at the teaching hospital. Discussion with consultant staff working in Leeds at the time indicated that on average a consultant would work five sessions in Leeds, with two or three sessions spent in peripheral hospitals and the remainder in private practice. It was on this basis that the 1948 figures were calculated. The data are not perfect but they do give what we believe is a fair indication of trends in the distribution of consultants in the Region.

13. For a discussion of these issues see J. Rickard, 'Per capita expenditure of English Area Health Authorities', *British Medical Journal*, 31 January 1976, pp. 299–300.
14. Stevens, *Medical Practice*.
15. C. E. Lindblom, 'The science of "muddling through"', *Public Administration Review*, 19 (1959) pp. 79–88.
16. G. Vickers, *The Art of Judgement* (London: Chapman and Hall, 1965).
17. *Report of the Joint Working Party on the Medical Staffing Structure in the Hospital Service* (London: HMSO, 1961).
18. Ministry of Health, Circular HM(64)94.
19. Ministry of Health, Circular HM(61)119.
20. *Medical Staffing Structure in Scottish Hospitals* (Edinburgh: HMSO, 1964) p. 7.
21. Ministry of Health, Circular HM(64)94.
22. *British Medical Journal Supplement*, 13 May 1967, pp. 93–6.
23. *British Medical Journal Supplement*, 16 March 1968, pp. 73–6; 22 February 1969, pp. 75–8; 6 December 1969, pp. 53–6; 28 August 1971, pp. 119–21; 19 August 1972, pp. 143–6.
24. *Royal Commission on Medical Education, 1965–1968*, Cmnd. 3569, (London: HMSO, 1968), ch. 3.
25. *Report of the Working Party on The Responsibilities of the Consultant Grade* (London: HMSO, 1969).
26. *British Medical Journal Supplement*, 6 July 1968, p. 8.
27. Ibid., p. 9.
28. *British Medical Journal*, 19 August 1972, p. 430.
29. Letter from the Chief Medical Officer to SAMOs, 8 August 1972.
30. This was the Crossman formula for redistributing financial resources, which was the precursor of the Resource Allocation Working Party (RAWP) formula.
31. Yorkshire Regional Health Authority, *Review of Health Services and Resources – Preparation of Outline Strategic Plans* (Harrogate, 1976), p. 150.
32. D. Owen, *In Sickness and In Health* (London: Quartet, 1976), p. 84.
33. M. A. R. Freeman, 'Possible future trends of Medical Staffing in the Hospitals of England and Wales', *British Medical Journal*, 6 December 1969, pp. 612–15.
34. In 1976 the Region was below the national average by 51 senior registrars and 92 registrars: Yorkshire RHA, *Regional Strategic Plan, 1977–1986* (Harrogate, 1977), p. 47.
35. *British Medical Journal*, 19 August 1972, p. 429.
36. Maynard and Walker, 'Doctor manpower'.
37. Freeman, 'Possible future trends', p. 612.
38. M. A. Elston, 'Medical autonomy: Challenge and response, in K. Barnard and K. Lee (eds.), *Conflicts in the National Health Service* (London: Croom Helm, 1977) p. 40.

Chapter 5

1. H. Eason, R. V. Clark and W. H. Harper, *Hospital Survey: The Hospital Services of the Yorkshire Area* (London: HMSO, 1945).
2. For planning purposes, the Board divided the Region into 13 hospital districts.
3. Ministry of Health Circular HM(57)86.
4. B. Isaacs, 'The training of a geriatric physician', *The Lancet*, 20 June 1964, pp. 1339–42.
5. *Annual Report of the Hospital Advisory Service for 1973* (London: HMSO, 1974) p. 23.
6. The Leeds Geriatric Service and its origins are described in a report published by the Leeds (A) and Leeds (B) HMCs in 1955.
7. Ministry of Health Circular HM(65)77.
8. Ibid.
9. A similar conclusion was reached by Greta Sumner and Randall Smith in *Planning Local Authority Services for the Elderly* (London: Allen and Unwin, 1969) pp. 115–17 and Chapter 20.
10. B. Robb (ed.), *Sans Everything – a Case to Answer* (London: Nelson, 1967).
11. *Findings and Recommendations following Enquiries into Allegations concerning the care of Elderly Patients in Certain Hospitals*, Cmnd. 3687, (London: HMSO, 1968).
12. The Board was able to find this money because it received a larger grant than expected from DHSS for the development of renal dialysis units, and through overprovision for staff.
13. At the beginning of each financial year the Board set aside a reserve to be used for employing extra staff and to be allocated to HMCs when these staff were taken on. There were usually funds remaining in these reserves at the end of the financial year.
14. These were non-recurring items which took up a large proportion of the additional allocations because part of these allocations arose from money which it had been planned to use to finance the revenue consequences of capital schemes, but which had been diverted to long-stay services because these schemes were completed late. As this money would be needed for its true purpose in later years it could not be used to finance developments which would be a permanent call on the Board's resources. This, of course, had the effect of limiting the continuing benefit to long-stay services of additional allocations.
15. For example, from 1972/1973 onwards an earmarked allocation was made specifically for capital improvements to geriatric services and services for the elderly with severe dementia. In 1973/1974 the Board received £610 000 under this arrangement.
16. In the *Annual Report of the Hospital Advisory Service for 1972* (London: HMSO, 1973) it was stated: 'At present the Teaching Hospitals provide poor examples of a comprehensive service for either mental illness or geriatrics and almost no service for the mentally handicapped. Although the reasons for this are historical, I am not satisfied that changes are

taking place sufficiently quickly. In particular, changes in attitudes seem to visiting teams to be occurring even more slowly at Teaching Hospitals than elsewhere and old attitudes are often particularly hard on the geriatrician.' (p. 15) And later: 'I am emphasising this matter of attitudes because there is little doubt that it underlies many of the difficulties now being experienced.'(p. 26)

17. K. Jones, *History of the Mental Health Services* (London: Routledge and Kegan Paul, 1972) p. 337.
18. *Report of the Committee of Enquiry into Allegations of Ill-Treatment of Patients and other irregularities at the Ely Hospital, Cardiff*, Cmnd. 3975 (London: HMSO, 1969).
19. Ibid., p. 127.
20. Ibid., p. 126.
21. Ibid., p. 98.
22. Ibid., p. 132.
23. R. Crossman, *The Diaries of a Cabinet Minister*, vol. 3, *Secretary of State for Social Services 1968–1970* (London: Hamilton and Cape, 1977) p. 413.
24. Ibid., p. 419.
25. Ibid., p. 456.
26. Ibid., p. 466.
27. Ibid., p. 455.
28. Ibid., p. 613.
29. The name 'Coleshill' came from the Coleshill Hospital at Birmingham where these units were developed by the Birmingham RHB. They later became known as 'Crossman' units because of the Secretary of State's interest in them.
30. *Annual Report of the Hospital Advisory Service for 1969/1970* (London: HMSO, 1971) p. 2.
31. Ibid., p. 5.
32. The HAS *Annual Report* for 1969/1970 included a letter from a ward sister to the Service pointing out improvements made to her hospital in preparation for a HAS team visit.
33. Legal proceedings against the patients at the Hospital followed.
34. K. Jones with J. Brown, W. J. Cunningham, J. Roberts and P. Williams, *Opening the Door* (London: Routledge and Kegan Paul, 1975) p. 20.
35. J. Pantall, *Training Project for Hospitals for the Mentally Handicapped* (1974, mimeo).
36. Ibid.
37. *Better Services for the Mentally Handicapped*, Cmnd. 4683, (London: HMSO, 1970).
38. Jones, *Opening the Door*, p. 180.
39. Ibid., p. 183.
40. *Report of the Farleigh Hospital Committee of Enquiry*, Cmnd. 4557, (London: HMSO, 1971); *Report of the Committee of Enquiry into Normansfield Hospital*, Cmnd. 7357 (London: HMSO, 1978).
41. *Report of the Royal Commission on the Laws Relating to Mental Illness and Mental Deficiency*, Cmnd. 169 (London: HMSO, 1957).

42. Quoted in Jones, *A History of the Mental Health Services*, p. 312. The title of the speech derives from the following description by Powell of mental hospitals: 'There they stand, isolated, majestic, imperious, brooded over by the gigantic water-tower and chimney combined, rising unmistakeable and daunting out of the countryside – the asylums which our forefathers built with such immense solidity.'
43. HM(61)25. G. C. Tooth and E. M. Brooke, 'Needs and beds: Trends in the mental health population and their effect on future planning', *The Lancet*, 1 April 1961, pp. 710–13.
44. Both quotations from HM(61)25.
45. Ibid.
46. *A Hospital Plan for England and Wales*, Cmnd. 1604 (London: HMSO, 1962) p. 11.
47. Ibid.
48. The survey was carried out by Dr Brian Ward and Dr Charles Gore of the RHB, and Dr Kathleen Jones and Dr Wallis Taylor of Manchester University. A summary of the results was published in *The Lancet*, 29 August 1964, pp. 457–60, as 'Needs and beds: A regional census of psychiatric hospital patients'.
49. These details came from an interview with Dr Arthur Bowen, the consultant psychiatrist mainly involved in the service, and from *York Mental Health Service First Report* (1953–7, mimeo).
50. A. Lindsey, *Socialised Medicine in England and Wales* (Chapel Hill: University of North Carolina Press, 1962) p. 318.
51. Circulars RHB(50)80 and RHB(51)84 recommended that a minimum of 20 per cent of capital expenditure should be allocated to mental health.
52. Report to the Board's General Purposes Committee, 8 April 1965.
53. The difference was accounted for by senile patients who tended to wander and who had to be kept in locked wards because of a shortage of nurses.
54. A. Clare, *Psychiatry in Dissent* (London: Tavistock Publications, 1976) p. 414.
55. HM(61)69. For a summary of the Working Party's Report see *Report of the Ministry of Health*, 1961, Cmnd. 1754 (London: HMSO, 1962) pp. 16–18.
56. *Interim Report of the Committee on Mentally Abnormal Offenders*, Cmnd. 5698 (London: HMSO, 1974).
57. Clare, *Psychiatry in Dissent*, p. 415.
58. W. A. L. Bowen, 'Need for inspection (or survey) of psychiatric hospital services' in H. Freeman (ed.), *Psychiatric Hospital Care* (London: Bailliere, Tindall and Cassell, 1965).
59. HAS *Annual Report*, 1969/1970, p. 17.
60. *Report of the Committee of Enquiry into Whittingham Hospital*, Cmnd. 4861 (London: HMSO, 1972).
61. Ibid., p. iii.
62. *The Facilities and Services of Mental Illness and Mental Handicap Hospitals in England and Wales 1973*, Statistical and Research Report Series No. 11 (London: HMSO, 1976). Statistics for 1974 showed some

improvement. Only five of the hospitals were below the minimum standards, the most common deficiencies again being personal cupboards and domestic staff: Statistical and Research Report Series No. 15 (London: HMSO, 1976).

63. The following five points have been adapted from the *Annual Report of the Hospital Advisory Service for 1972* (London: HMSO, 1973) pp. 3–4.

64. *Report of the Committee of Enquiry into St. Augustine's Hospital, Chartham, Canterbury* (South East Thames RHA, 1976) p. 81.

65. *Annual Report of the Hospital Advisory Service for 1975* (London: HMSO, 1976) p. v.

66. HAS *Annual Report*, 1972, p. 6.

67. *Annual Report of the Hospital Advisory Service for 1973* (London: HMSO, 1974) p. 11.

68. Ibid., foreword.

69. D. Gould, 'Sickness in the health service', *New Statesman*, 12 September 1973, pp. 301–3.

70. *Better Services for the Mentally Ill*, Cmnd. 6233 (London: HMSO, 1975).

71. K. Jones, 'Mental health administration: Reflections from the British experience', *Administration in Mental Health*, vol. 4[2], Spring 1977, p. 6.

Chapter 6

1. The 'theory' of disjointed incrementalism is outlined in D. Braybrooke and C. E. Lindblom, *A Strategy of Decision* (London: Collier Macmillan,1963).

2. E. E. Schattschneider, *The Semisovereign People* (New York: Holt, Rinehart and Winston, 1960) p. 38.

3. H. Eason, R. V. Clark and W. H. Harper, *Hospital Survey: The Hospital Services of the Yorkshire Area* (London: HMSO, 1945).

4. A report to the Board in 1953 by the SAMO noted Craig's refusal to 'accept the repeated earnest invitations from several quarters to become a member of the Paediatric Panel, and thus give his paediatric colleagues and the medical staff of the Regional Board the benefit of his wide experience'.

5. P. Bachrach and M. S. Baratz, *Power and Poverty* (New York: Oxford University Press, 1970) p. 44.

6. G. Allison, *Essence of Decision* (Boston: Little Brown, 1971).

7. R. R. Alford, *Health Care Politics* (University of Chicago Press, 1975).

Chapter 7

1. H. Eckstein, *The English Health Service* (Cambridge, Mass: Harvard University Press, 1958) p. 193.

2. *Report on Co-operation between Hospital, Local Authority and General Practitioner Services* (London: HMSO, 1952).

3. *Report of the Committee of Enquiry into the Cost of the NHS*, Cmd. 9663, (London: HMSO, 1956) p. 236.

4. See Chapter 5.
5. *Report of the Committee of Enquiry into the Cost of the NHS.*
6. J. E. Tibbitt, *Collaboration Between Health and Social Work Services: Transactions at the Interface* (mimeo, 1976).
7. D. Towell, *Approaches to Joint Care Planning* (mimeo, 1977).
8. *Report of the Maternity Services Committee* (London: HMSO, 1959).
9. For a fuller discussion of these arrangements, see Chapter 5.
10. *Health and Welfare: The Development of Community Care*, Cmnd. 1973, (London: HMSO, 1963).
11. B. Davies, *Social Needs and Resources in Local Services* (London: Michael Joseph, 1968) p. 206.
12. *Health and Welfare* (1963), p. 2.
13. Ibid., p. iii.
14. *Health and Welfare: The Development of Community Care*, Cmnd. 3022, (London: HMSO, 1966), p. 26.
15. J. A. G. Griffith, *Central Departments and Local Authorities* (London: Allen and Unwin, 1966) p. 515.
16. K. Judge, *Rationing Social Services* (London: Heinemann, 1978) chapter 4.
17. Griffith, *Central Departments and Local Authorities*, p. 467.
18. R. G. S. Brown, *The Management of Welfare* (London: Fontana, 1975), pp. 131–4. Brown's analysis applies to the 1972 ten year plans but is equally applicable to the earlier versions.
19. *Report of the Committee on Local Authority and Allied Personal Social Services*, Cmnd. 3703, (London: HMSO, 1968).
20. P. Hall, *Reforming the Welfare* (London: Heinemann, 1976) p. 109.
21. *Better Services for the Mentally Handicapped* Cmnd. 4683, (London: HMSO, 1971).
22. K. Jones with J. Brown, W. J. Cunningham, J. Roberts and P. Williams, *Opening the Door* (London: Routledge and Kegan Paul, 1975) p. 180.
23. RHB (49) 132.
24. See especially R. Stevens, *Medical Practice in Modern England* (New Haven: Yale University Press, 1966).
25. *The Field of Work of the Family Doctor*, The Gillie Report (London: HMSO, 1963) p. 63.
26. See Chapter 4.
27. *Report of the Committee on General Practice within the NHS* (London: HMSO, 1954).
28. *The Field Work of the Family Doctor.*
29. Ibid., p. 47.
30. Ibid. These difficulties were even more apparent at York where the Board first tried to launch the pilot scheme. The HMC was only prepared to allocate beds for use by GPs in an isolation hospital, and this proved "unrealistic and unacceptable" to the Board.
31. *Royal Commission on Medical Education*, Cmnd. 3569, (London: HMSO, 1968).
32. K. Jones, 'Mental health administration: Reflections from the British experience', *Administration in Mental Health*, vol. 4[2] (Spring 1977).

33. This paragraph draws on the work of G. T. Allison, *Essence of Decision* (Boston: Little Brown, 1971).

Chapter 8

1. *Eighth Report from the Expenditure Committee*, Session 1971/1972, Relationship of Expenditure to Needs, HC 515, Services for the Elderly, Memorandum submitted by DHSS.
2. Ibid.
3. Ibid., Minutes of Evidence, 23 May 1972.
4. J. E. Powell, *A New Look at Medicine and Politics* (London: Pitman, 1966), p. 56.
5. Richard Crossman, *A Politician's View of Health Service Planning* (University of Glasgow, 1972) p. 10.
6. *The Future Structure of the National Health Service* (London: HMSO, 1970).
7. Quoted in *The Report of the Committee of Enquiry into the Cost of the National Health Service,* Cmd. 9663 (London: HMSO, 1956) p. 79.
8. Ibid.
9. Ibid., p. 83.
10. See the criticisms of the Acton Society Trust in *Creative Leadership in a State Service* (1959).
11. Interview with G. Wilson, Assistant Secretary, Ministry of Health, during the 1960s, with responsibility for hospital planning and building.
12. *Report of the Committee of Enquiry into Allegations of Ill-Treatment of Patients and other irregularities at the Ely Hospital, Cardiff,* Cmnd. 3975 (London: HMSO, 1969).
13. D. Owen, *In Sickness and In Health* (London: Quartet, 1976) p. 8.
14. K. Judge, *Rationing Social Services* (London: Heinemann, 1978) Chapter 4, contains a useful discussion of central-local relations in the personal social services.
15. Estimates Committee (Sub-Committee B), *Hospital Building in Great Britain*, Part of Minutes of Evidence, 8 December 1969, Session 1969/1970, HC 59-i.
16. See Chapter 4.
17. R. G. S. Brown, 'The course of a circular – a study of reactions to HM(62) 1', *The Hospital*, June 1962, pp. 371–4.
18. R. Stewart and J. Sleeman, 'Continuously under review', *Occasional Papers on Social Administration*, no. 20 (London: Bell, 1967).
19. R. G. S. Brown, *Reorganising the National Health Service* (Oxford: Blackwell and Robertson, 1979) p. 11.
20. This was a grade established in 1948 as a temporary measure for those doctors with the experience but not the qualifications to be graded as consultants. Regular reviews of the doctors in SHMO posts were undertaken right up until the early 1970s. Although conceived as a temporary measure, new appointments to the grade were made until 1964 when it was finally closed.
21. Crossman, *A Politician's View*, p. 13.

22. *Report of the Committee of Enquiry in to the Cost of the National Health Service*, p. 83.
23. *The Administrative Structure of the Medical and Related Services in England and Wales* (London: HMSO, 1968) pp. 9–10.
24. J. A. G. Griffith, *Central Departments and Local Authorities* (London: Allen and Unwin, 1966) pp. 515–23.
25. P. Self, *Administrative Theories and Politics* (London: Allen and Unwin, 1972) p. 98.
26. *Local Government Finance: Report of the Committee of Enquiry*, Cmnd. 6453 (London: HMSO, 1976).
27. Crossman, *A Politician's View*, p. 22.
28. Expenditure Committee (Employment and Social Services Sub-Committee) Minutes of Evidence, 31st March 1971, Session 1970/1971, HC 323 ii.
29. R. Klein, 'Policy problems and policy perceptions in the National Health Service', *Policy and Politics*, vol. 2[3], (1974) pp. 219–36; R. Klein, 'Policy making in the National Health Service' *Political Studies*, Vol. xxii [1] (1974) pp. 1–14.

Chapter 9

1. R. G. S. Brown, *The Changing National Health Service* (London: Routledge and Kegan Paul, 1973); B. Watkin, *The National Health Service: The First Phase* (London: George Allen and Unwin, 1978).
2. J. E. Powell, *A New Look at Medicine and Politics* (London: Pitman, 1966) p. 16.
3. P. Draper, G. Best and J. Dennis, *Health, Money and the National Health Service* (London: Unit for the Study of Health Policy, 1976) p. 12.
4. Abel-Smith has put it like this: 'Britain's health service was once claimed to be the envy of the world. Without doubt it is the envy of the world's finance ministers.' See 'The Cost of Health Services', *New Society*, vol. 49 (1979) no. 875, p. 76.
5. A. Cochrane, *Effectiveness and Efficiency: Random Reflections on Health Services* (London: Nuffield Provincial Hospitals Trust, 1972).
6. See, for example, A. Culyer, *Need and the National Health Service* (London: Martin Robertson, 1976).
7. See, for example, D. Owen, 'Clinical freedom and professional freedom', *The Lancet*, 8 May 1976.
8. As an example, see the essays contained in C. Cox and A. Mead (eds.), *A Sociology of Medical Practice* (London: Collier–Macmillan, 1975).
9. I. Illich, *Limits to Medicine* (London: Marion Boyars, 1976).
10. R. G. S. Brown, *Reorganising the National Health Service* (Oxford: Blackwell and Robertson, 1979) pp. 199–200.
11. Ibid., p. 212. See also G. Godber, 'Regional devolution and the National Health Service' in E. Craven (ed.), *Regional Devolution and Social Policy* (London: Macmillan, 1975).
12. Richard Crossman, *A Politician's View of Health Service Planning* (University of Glasgow Press, 1972) p. 10.

13. See DHSS, *The NHS Planning System* (London: HMSO, June 1976).
14. DHSS, *Draft Guide to Planning in the NHS* (London: HMSO, 1975).
15. DHSS, *Priorities for Health and Personal Social Services in England* (London: HMSO, 1976); *The Way Forward* (London: HMSO, 1977); and circulars HC(78)12 and HC(79)9.
16. D. Towell, 'Making reorganisation work' in K. Barnard and K. Lee, *Conflicts in the National Health Service* (London: Croom Helm, 1977), p. 168.
17. Brown, *Reorganising the National Health Service*, pp. 213–14.
18. S. Dimmock, 'Participation or control? The workers' involvement in management', in Barnard and Lee, *Conflicts in the National Health Service*, p. 121.
19. R. Alford, *Health Care Politics* (University of Chicago Press, 1975).
20. A. Wildavsky, *Speaking Truth to Power. The Art and Craft of Policy Analysis* (Boston: Little Brown, 1979).
21. H. Heclo and A. Wildavsky, *The Private Government of Public Money* (London: Macmillan, 1974); J. Edwards and R. Batley, *The Politics of Positive Discrimination* (London: Tavistock, 1978). Much of the argument in this section is based on C. J. Ham, 'Approaches to the study of social policy making', *Policy and Politics*, vol. 8, no. 1 (January 1980).
22. Alford, *Health care Politics*, p. 17.
23. G. Vickers, *The Art of Judgement* (London: Chapman and Hall, 1965) p. 67.
24. K. Young, '"Values" in the policy process', *Policy and Politics*, Vol. 5[3], (1977) p. 3.
25. K. Young and L. Mills, 'Understanding the "assumptive worlds" of governmental actors: Issues and approaches' (mimeo, 1978) pp. 7–8.
26. Ibid.
27. S. Lukes, *Power: A Radical View* (London: Macmillan, 1974) p. 41.
28. R. Klein, 'Policy making in the National Health Service', *Political Studies*, Vol. xxii[i] (1974) p. 1.

Index